Cleveland's Bitter Pill

Cleveland's Bitter Pill

A Diagnosis of Injured Title Dreams and Die-Hard Fans

Joseph Congeni, MD
with Thomas Bacher

Ringtaw Books
Akron, Ohio

19 18 17 16 15 5 4 3 2 1

ISBN: 978-1-935603-50-4 (paperback)

LIBRARY OF CONGRESS CATALOGING-IN-PUBLICATION DATA
Congeni, Joseph.
Cleveland's bitter pill : a diagnosis of injured title dreams and die-hard fans / Joseph Congeni, MD, with Thomas Bacher.
pages cm
ISBN 978-1-935603-50-4 (pbk. : alk. paper)
1. Sports—Ohio—Cleveland—History. 2. Sports injuries. I. Bacher, Thomas. II. Title.
GV584.5.C58C66 2015
796.771'32—dc23

2014044295

∞ The paper used in this publication meets the minimum requirements of ANSI / NISO Z39.48–1992 (Permanence of Paper).

Cover: (Left to right) Ray Chapman (Library of Congress, Prints & Photographs Division, LC-DIG-ggbain-27249), Ernie Davis (Photographs and clippings of Ernie Davis, University Archives, Syracuse University Libraries), and LeBron James (AP Photo/Mark Duncan).

Cleveland's Bitter Pill was designed and typeset in Minion with Helvetica display by Amy Freels, with assistance from Samantha Pasa, and printed on sixty-pound natural and bound by Bookmasters of Ashland, Ohio.

Contents

Acknowledgments

I would like to thank my wife Karen and my six children, Anthony, Brenna, Serafina, Francesca, Lucia, and Dominic for their time and patience while I was working on this book.

I would also like to extend my gratitude to David Clark, an English instructor at Cristo Rey Columbus High School, Columbus, Ohio, for researching and developing the idea for this book.

Introduction

Cleveland fans love their sports teams. The relationship, however, has been a painful one. After all, the last time the city celebrated a championship was in 1964, when the Browns beat the Baltimore Colts. That victory capped a fantastic era from 1946 until the early 1960s that brought home eight championships in the All-American Football Conference and the National Football League. Through 1965, the Browns played in thirteen championship games, losing five times. In a twenty-year span, the Browns were championship game contenders 65 percent of the time.

The other major sport team during that era, the Cleveland Indians, had a great deal of success, too. The Indians won the World Series in 1948 and appeared in the World Series in 1954. The team finished second in the American League in 1951, 1952, 1953, 1955, 1956, and 1959.

After the 1964 championship, the loyalty of Cleveland fans has been tested beyond comprehension. Browns fans have had to endure "Red Right 88," "The Drive," "The Fumble," and Modell's "Move." Indians fans have had to be strong enough to overcome the "The Curse of Rocky Colavito," and World Series losses in 1995 and 1997, the latter being all the more painful because the team's ace reliever couldn't hold a one-run lead in the ninth inning of game seven. The Cavaliers, the newest of the city's professional sports franchises, were at times almost comical when they started out in 1970. However, as the team progressed, Cavaliers fans have had to withstand disappointments of their own. In 1989, "The Shot" by Michael Jordan decimated the hearts of the Cleveland faithful and cost the Cavaliers a possible championship run. Although LeBron James has now returned to Cleveland, his "Decision" to take his talents to Miami left the city in mourning.

In the wake of all this despair, Cleveland sports fans have grown more passionate and rabid over the years. Local radio sports talk shows fill the airwaves and fans are not shy about expressing their opinions. When the new Cleveland Indians ballpark, Jacobs Field (now Progressive Field) opened, fans responded with 455 consecutive sellouts from 1995 to 2001. Despite the economic downturn and rooting for a team that hasn't won five games since 2007, Browns home games have not been blacked out. What drives the Cleveland fan to hope against all odds? Why does generation after generation still support the local clubs? What binds the area sports rooters into a "Fraternity of Misery"? Perhaps Cleveland fans come together to fight off the outsiders. Area supporters can criticize their own teams, but they won't tolerate any criticism from rival fans, including Steelers, Yankees, Celtics, or Heat followers. Maybe the hardworking ethic in and around Cleveland allows fans to take their yearly lumps because they know next year will be better, even if next year brings much of the same.

Sometimes, Cleveland fans feel cursed. No matter how far one of their teams might go, a dark cloud always seems to follow and a storm denies the fans their championship. Cleveland fans live week to week and even day to day. Earlier results mean nothing and rooters' impatience can lead to quick dismissals of coaches and general managers. Owners can't escape fans' wrath, either. Cleveland teams rarely land high-salaried free agents and lose their own free agents to higher-bidding organizations. Fans have to reacquaint themselves with new rosters continually. This lack of stability is best illustrated by the facts that since 1999 the Browns have had twenty starting quarterback, the Indians have had seven managers, and the Cavaliers have had seven head coaches. The Cleveland Camelot has turned into Cleveland Chaos.

National media outlets like to provide fodder for fans' ire. Cleveland is the "mistake on the lake" and that moniker plays out in dismal professional sports teams. Except in a few rare instances, ineptitude leads to ineffectiveness and the cycle is continuous. However, national pundits don't quite understand the Cleveland fan. Cleveland rooters tend to see the bright side and relish in the small victories that galvanize Cleveland's fan base.

Cavs fans became Mavs supporters and soaked up Dallas's victory over the LeBron-led Miami Heat in the 2011 NBA Finals. In December 2009, on a bitterly cold Thursday evening, the Browns defeated Ben Roethlisberger and the Steelers, knocking them out of the playoffs. The victory ended a twelve-game losing streak against Pittsburgh and local fans celebrated the outcome as if it were a Super Bowl triumph. With a roster of very few stars, the Cleveland Indians managed to make baseball's one-game playoff in 2013. Even after "The Decision," fans recovered and began speculating about the next superstar the Cavaliers could draft.

The wariness of Cleveland fans runs deep. In June 1948, the year the Indians would go on to win the World Series, a story in the *Cleveland Plain Dealer* by Sports Editor Gordon Cobbledick pointed out that Indians fans were "... afraid to believe this year may be different," because they had been disappointed so many times recently. In 1954, at a point in the season when the Indians had already won 109 games, some fans booed the team after the September loss to the Chicago White Sox. A local columnist wryly pointed out the team had, after all, lost 41 games. For area fans, any loss might be the first in a series leading to disaster.

Fans booed Brian Sipe in 1982, only two years after he was named the MVP of the NFL. In 1904, thousands of Cleveland fans contended that the baseball team (then named the Naps) didn't want to win a pennant because it would be disastrous for the club and its finances—a great rationale for failure (*Plain Dealer,* February 20, 1909). The year after Frank Ryan helped win the NFL Championship for the Cleveland Browns, fans jeered him and questioned his leadership skills. And to add insult to injury, the local media took time to point out that T-shirts of Super Joe Charboneau and the Kardiac

Kids could be found on the clearance tables of local department stores after the dreams of a possible championship turned into cellar dwelling.

However, even with disaster lurking in the corners of the area's professional sporting venues, fans don't really give up. Browns Backers Worldwide boasts over 340 chapters and over 90,000 members. It seems moving elsewhere can strengthen fans' commitments to their home teams. Cleveland is a sports town built on the enduring hope and indestructible dreams of its passionate fans. Wearing emotions on their collective sleeves, fans can take heartbreak as long as they experience thrills along the way. Every Clevelander knows the shining championship moment is still attainable.

In the 1950s, Cleveland ranked as the seventh largest city in the country. By 1970, it was tenth and in 2010, the city had dropped to sixteenth. Faced with putting together smaller-market teams, the Browns, Cavaliers, and Indians don't have the luxury of having deep rosters. From torn rotator cuffs to torn knee ligaments, from sprained ankles to sprained backs, and from broken legs to broken arms, Cleveland's bitter pill has taken some of its best athletes and immobilized them at inopportune times. Shaq gave fans his inside dominance and his ailing thumb in 2010. Herb Score was a blazing left-hander until he took a line drive to the face in 1957. When the Las Vegas oddsmakers picked the Browns to win the Super Bowl in 1988, Bernie Kosar's arm injury derailed championship aspirations. These are just a few of the stories that follow.

Cleveland Indians

1915–present American League
Last World Series Title—1920

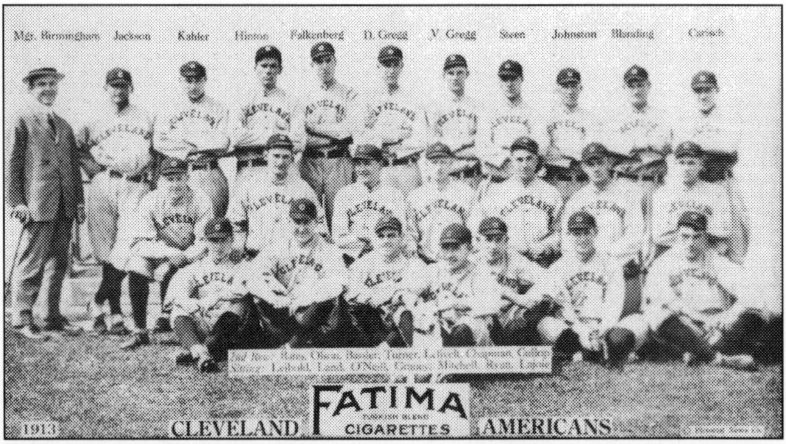

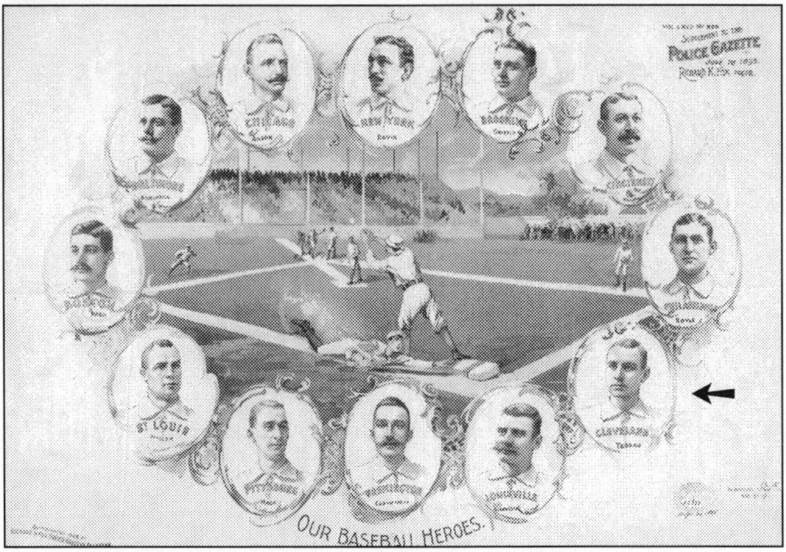

(Top) Cleveland Naps, 1913 (Library of Congress, Prints & Photographs Division, LC-DIG-bbc-2077f)

(Bottom) Portraits of the captains of the twelve baseball teams in the National League including Oliver W. "Patsy" Tebeau of the Cleveland Spiders, 1895. (Library of Congress, Prints & Photographs Division, LC-DIG-ppmsca-18403)

In 1871 and 1872, Cleveland fielded a team named the Forest Citys in the first professional baseball league in America. When the National League formed, Cleveland participated from 1879 through 1884 as the Cleveland Blues. The team moved to the American Association for the 1887 and 1888 seasons. The Cleveland Infants played for one year (1890) in the short-lived Players League. By 1889, Cleveland's National League team was known as the Spiders. Ignominiously, the 1899 Cleveland Spiders finished with the worst record ever in professional baseball. The team won 20 games and lost a stunning 134. The most wins any starting pitcher registered that year were four.

Even when Cleveland teams weren't part of one of the major leagues, local baseball was still popular. Fans must have truly gotten their money's worth during a May 17, 1870, contest between the Forest Citys and the Atlantics. By the end of the fifth inning, the Forest Citys were ahead 132–1, having belted out 180 hits, 101 of them singles.

On April 21, 1901, the Cleveland Blues, of the newly formed American Baseball League, hosted Chicago to inaugurate play in the circuit that would rival the decades-old National League. Cleveland lost 8–2. The team changed its name the following year to the Bronchos and again in 1903 to the Naps, for their star player Napoleon Lajoie. When Lajoie left after the 1914 season, local sportswriters temporarily chose the name Indians "as the club may so conduct itself during the present season as to earn some other cognomen which may be more appropriate" (*Plain Dealer,* January 17, 1915). In part, the name was a throwback to 1897. A Native American, Louis Sockalexis, was a fabulous rookie on the 1897 team and fans began referring to the team as the Indians. Unfortunately, midway through the season Sockalexis's career plummeted after the inebriated star jumped out of a second-story window and broke his ankle.

A Pitcher Felled by the White Plague

Adrian C. "Addie" "The Maestro of Twirlology" Joss

Born: 1880 Died: 1911
Cleveland Bluebirds and
Cleveland Naps: 1902–10
Position: Pitcher
Jersey Number: N/A (Numbers were not worn at this time. In 1916, the Cleveland Indians were the first team to employ numbers, which were affixed to the jersey's left sleeve.)

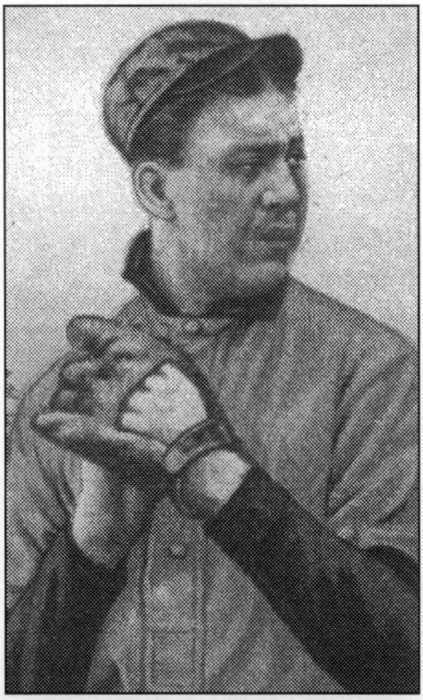

Addie Joss, American Tobacco Company Trading Card, early 1900s (Library of Congress, Prints & Photographs Division, LC-DIG-bbc-0923f)

SYMPTOMS

Addie Joss was born in 1880 in Woodland, Wisconsin, and went on to play baseball with several semiprofessional clubs. In the spring of 1898, Charles Strobel, owner of Strobel Aviation and the Toledo club of the Interstate League, signed the pitcher. Joss developed his skills with Toledo before moving to Cleveland in 1902.

In 1907, Joss posted a league-leading 27–11 record. Nonetheless, the Naps finished at 77–75 and in fifth place. The following year, Joss led the league with a stellar 1.16 ERA and pitched a perfect game, throwing only seventy-four pitches during the contest. By September 22, the Naps had overtaken Detroit for the top spot in the American League, and the race was destined to go down to the wire. In the end, Cleveland and Detroit tied with 90 victories, but Detroit only lost 63 games to Cleveland's 64 (rainouts were not always replayed). Detroit went on to the World Series and lost to the Chicago Cubs.

Joss seemed set to lead the team again in 1909, but his record fell to 14–13 and his strikeout numbers for nine innings also declined. The following season, Joss developed what the *Plain Dealer* described as "a ligament torn loose over the elbow of his pitching arm" (June 15, 1910). He tried to pitch but was ineffective, finishing with a 5–5 record, and after August didn't pitch for the rest of the season.

Joss returned to spring training in 1911 and pronounced himself fit enough to be part of the starting rotation. But in early April, after he suddenly fainted at the Naps' Chattanooga training camp, the team sent him back home to Toledo. The Cleveland team physician Dr. M. H. Castle visited him on April 13 and called the Tribe hurler a very sick man. Joss had initially suffered a bout of pleurisy, but was now showing signs of possible brain hemorrhaging. The next day Joss passed away from tuberculous meningitis at the age of thirty-one. The team refused to play a scheduled game with the Tigers in Detroit and made the trip to Toledo for the funeral.

Among the telegrams that Joss's widow received was one from Mr. and Mrs. Ty Cobb. "Please accept our deepest sympathies in your present bereavement. The shock was terrible to us. He numbered his friends by his acquaintances. We cannot find words to express feelings as we should" (*Plain Dealer*, April 6, 1911).

In 1978, Joss was elected to the Baseball Hall of Fame by the veteran's committee.

PATIENT HISTORY

"Joss sort of hid the ball on you. One moment, you'd be squinting at a long graceful windup and the next instant, out of nowhere, the ball was hopping across the plate—and a lot of us standing flat-footed with our bats glued to our shoulders!"
—Bobby Wallace, Baseball Hall of Famer

"There is not a star pitcher in this country today but had to take some terrific beatings before he acquired the wisdom that made him a star."
—Addie Joss

"I agree with Addie Joss when he said that pitching was the biggest part of the game. If I had had Vean Gregg to work along with Addie back in 1908 we would have played the Cubs for the world's pennant, but one star pitcher rarely wins a pennant, especially if that star is a man who needs at least three days in between his games."
—Nap Lajoie, Cleveland manager and Baseball Hall of Famer

DIAGNOSIS

Addie Joss's tragic death came over a decade before Ray Chapman's death as the result of getting hit by a pitch. While Chapman always seemed to represent Tribe injury misfortune, Joss could easily have been the first sign of bad luck—a very rare and rapidly spreading form of meningitis struck the pitcher down in his prime. Joss was the dominant pitcher of the early 1900s; without Joss, the Naps drifted out of contention.

SECOND OPINION

The Naps might have overcome the loss of Joss if Vean Gregg had stayed healthy. Gregg was a six-foot-two and 180-pound southpaw who had a devastating curve ball. As a twenty-six-year-old rookie for the 1911 Cleveland Naps, Gregg won 23 games and led the American League with a 1.80 ERA. Both Ty Cobb and Eddie Collins called him the best left-hander in the league. In his first three major league campaigns, Gregg won at least 20 games, the only twentieth-century pitcher to do so. Unfortunately, Gregg developed arm trouble and was eventually traded to Boston. Gregg is attributed with coining the phrase "dust him off" as a more civil way of indicating that a pitcher might bean (throw close to) an opposing batter to deter the batter from leaning over the plate.

TREATMENT

Tuberculous meningitis (TBM), the most common form of central nervous system tuberculosis, is caused by Mycobacterium tuberculosis (M. tuberculosis), which usually spreads to the brain from another site in the body. Symptoms can include low-grade fever, malaise, headache, dizziness, vomiting, and/or personality changes that may persist for a few weeks, after which patients can then develop more severe headache, altered mental status, stroke, hydrocephalus (buildup of fluid inside the skull that leads to brain swelling), and cranial neuropathies (diseases or malfunctions of the nerves). When allowed to progress without treatment, coma and death almost always ensue.

According to the World Health Organization, tuberculosis (TB) is second only to HIV/AIDS as the greatest killer worldwide due to a single infectious agent. Over 95 percent of TB deaths occur in low- and middle-income countries. There were 569 deaths from TB in 2010 in the United States, as compared to 776 deaths in 2000. (In the early 1900s, an estimated 110,000 Americans died each year from tuberculosis.) The lower rate of TB occurrence and death in the United States can be attributed to early testing, primarily using the TB Skin Test (Mantoux Test), a test that has been in use for over a hundred years.

With appropriate antibiotic treatment TB can be cured in most people. Treatment usually involves taking several antibiotic drugs (e.g., isoniazid and rifampicin) for at least six months and sometimes for as long as twelve months. Multi-drug-resistant (MDR) TB has now become an issue, with 650,000 people infected globally in 2010 as reported by the WHO. Treatment of MDR TB includes a regiment of several different antibiotics, but between as many as six of every ten patients will die from the disease.

INCIDENTAL FINDINGS

In the early days of Cleveland baseball, games were played at League Park, which was built in 1891 at the corner of Dunham Street (later East 66th) and Lexington Avenue. The original capacity of the wooden structure was 9,000. Renovated over the years, the new and improved concrete League Park reopened in 1910, capable of accommodating up to 24,414 fans.

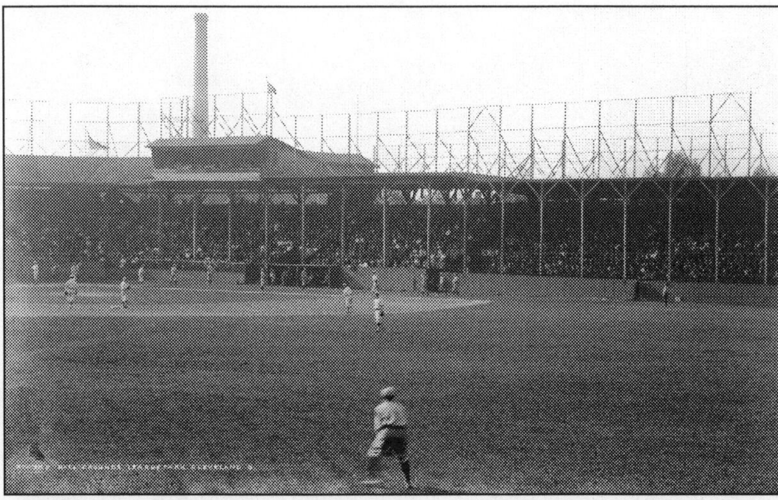

League Park, Cleveland, early 1900s (Library of Congress, Prints & Photographs Division, LC-DIG-det-4a22969)

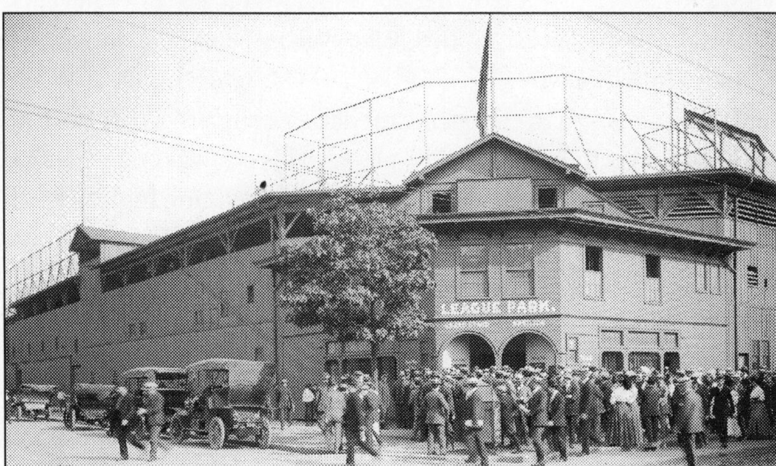

League Park entrance, Cleveland, early 1900s (Library of Congress, Prints & Photographs Division, LC-DIG-det-4a18626)

A Death on the Diamond

Raymond Johnson "Ray" "Chappie" Chapman

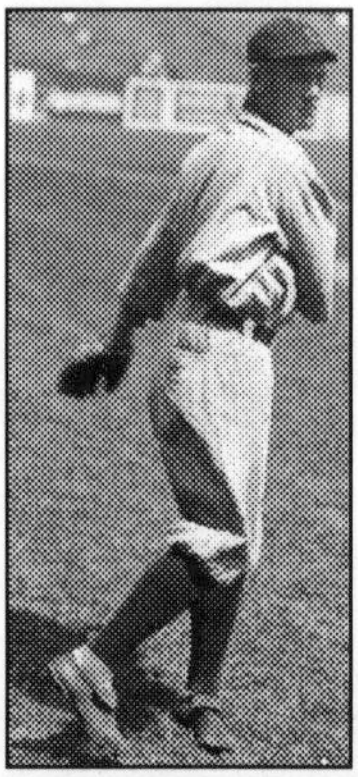

Born: 1891 Died: 1920
Cleveland Naps: 1912–14
Cleveland Indians: 1915–20
Position: Shortstop
Jersey Number: 2

Ray Chapman, 1919 (Library of Congress, Prints & Photographs Division, LC-DIG-ggbain-27249)

SYMPTOMS

Ray Chapman played his entire career as a shortstop for the Cleveland Naps and Indians. Over his nine years with the Tribe he batted .278. By all accounts, he was a popular player and was well liked by teammates and fans. In August 1920, Chapman's club was leading the New York Yankees by two games in the loss column. The Indians topped the American League in team batting and team fielding averages, and fans were hopeful that a pennant would grace League Park.

On Monday August 16, the Tribe was in New York to face the Yankees in a key series. The Yanks had just returned from Washington and had lost the last game in that series by a 6–4 margin. Carl Mays, probably the most disliked player of his era, was on the mound for the home team. He had the reputation of sending high fastballs at batters to back them off the plate. Chapman's crouching-over-the-plate style had made him prone to being hit by pitches.

Chapman led off the top of the fifth inning at the Polo Grounds. Mays threw a fastball that "sailed." Chapman seemed to freeze and the ball struck him on the skull with a crack that was heard around the stadium. Newspapers of the day reported that Chapman dropped, unconscious, and the home plate umpire asked if there was a physician available, as Chapman was bleeding from the ear. The Indians' shortstop attempted to get up and walk off the field, but his knees buckled and he had to be assisted by two teammates, first to the clubhouse and then to an ambulance. Chapman was taken to a hospital and he lost consciousness enroute. He never woke up, and died after surgery early the next morning. His body was transported back to Cleveland and he is buried in Lake View Cemetery.

The reasons that Chapman failed to get out of the way varied; his front cleat got stuck in the dirt, he was expecting a curve ball, he lost sight of the ball in the day's twilight. Several clubs called for Mays to be banned for the rest of the season. Mays said that the ball was scuffed and the umpires were to blame. Two umpires responded by saying that no "pitcher in the American League resorted to trickery more than Carl Mays." Earlier that year, baseball had outlawed the spitball, mud ball, emery ball, and all other trick pitches, but enforcement was difficult at best. Mays was allowed to stay with the Yankees and played until 1929.

Initially, the Indians replaced Chapman with second-year shortstop Harry Lunte. However, Lunte pulled a leg muscle in early September and Joe Sewell, a player from the team's New Orleans minor league affiliate, was called up. Sewell, who would go on to have a Hall of Fame career, said he played that season with Chapman's spirit. The rest of the Indians adopted the spirit as well and went on to capture their first ever American League pennant. The Indians then captured the 1920 World Series, beating the Brooklyn Dodgers in the best-of-nine Fall Classic by 5 games to 2. The series was notable for an unassisted triple play pulled off by Tribe second baseman Bill Wambsganss.

PATIENT HISTORY

> "To the small boy, to the grown man, to the aged, he was the clean wholesome, gentle comrade."
> —William A Seullen, chancellor of the Cleveland Diocese

"Down through the years, he team-worked for victory, never sulking, always optimistic"
—*The Providence News*

"Chapman's is one more proof of the great truth to win real success we must attain character."
—Association Men (YMCA)

DIAGNOSIS

Ray Chapman's death brought dark clouds that covered Cleveland fans like a gloomy Ohio winter. Chapman's untimely demise might have cemented the injury saga that has haunted Cleveland teams to this day. After all, Chapman was on top of the world. He had married Kathleen Daly, the daughter of the very wealthy president of the East Ohio Gas Company. Kathleen was pregnant with the couple's first child (a daughter who would be named Rae) when Chapman got beaned. The infielder had planned to retire from the game after the 1920 season and become a businessman.

Chapman's family didn't thrive after his death. Chapman's bride eventually remarried and moved to Los Angeles, but in 1928 also died young. Rae Marie, Chapman's daughter, died a year later of measles. The string of related deaths makes the Chapman incident and its impact on Cleveland seem even more believable. Does Ray's ghost still haunt the city on Lake Erie?

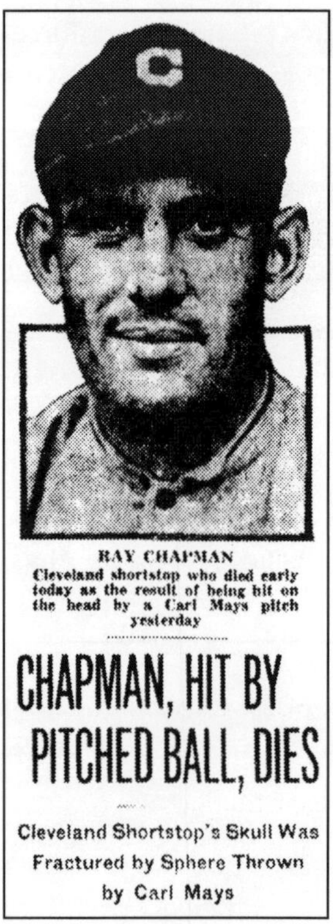

RAY CHAPMAN
Cleveland shortstop who died early today as the result of being hit on the head by a Carl Mays pitch yesterday

CHAPMAN, HIT BY PITCHED BALL, DIES

Cleveland Shortstop's Skull Was Fractured by Sphere Thrown by Carl Mays

Headline from the *Evening Public Ledger*, Philadelphia, PA, August 17, 1920.

SECOND OPINION

Chapman's death was untimely, but the Indians found a stellar replacement in Joe Sewell. In fact, Sewell would bat .320 during his Cleveland career, 42 points higher than Chapman. Sewell was also a slightly better fielder.

Poor Tribe pitching and the rise of the Babe Ruth Yankees ended up derailing the Tribe's hopes for another World Series crown. The 1920 season was highlighted by Jim "Sarge" Bagby's 31-win season, a mark he never approached again. The following two seasons, he won 14 and 4 games, respectively. By 1923, the Tribe's ERA had dropped to seventh of the eight teams in the American League. The Bronx Bombers finished first in the American League six times from 1921 through 1929 and won the World Series three times.

TREATMENT

Traumatic brain injuries (TBI) include concussions (see medical illustration, page 295) as well as brain bleeds. Bleeding in the brain is much less common in sport-related injuries than concussions. Brain bleeds can include an actual laceration or tear of the brain tissue, but more frequently appear in the form of a hematoma, which is a collection of blood in or around the brain. A hematoma often leads to increased pressure within the skull, causing symptoms like paralysis, weakness on one side of the body, or a blown pupil that fails to respond to light. In extreme cases, pressure can lead to a slower heart rate, an increase in blood pressure, and slowed breathing. These are life-threatening symptoms.

Better imaging techniques in the last two decades have helped medical professionals make more timely diagnoses and save lives. A CT (computed tomography) scan is generally the most useful tool for a rapid diagnosis. Lifesaving interventions or treatments include intubation, use of a ventilator, and the use of strong medicines to rapidly reduce the intracranial pressure. Surgery may also be necessary to decompress or reduce the swelling in the brain. Emergency medical teams on the sidelines are trained to look for and respond to these rare but life-threatening brain injuries at today's sporting events.

INCIDENTAL FINDINGS

Chapman was known to lean in at the plate, but ballplayers of that era understood that pitchers wouldn't respect them if they gave way to the bean ball. Ty Cobb painted the picture clearly:

> If you step back and fail to stand up to the plate on the next pitch after a close shave, all the twirlers in the league are soon on you. One tells another. Several of the pitchers tried this trick on me when I was first breaking into fast company. I made up my mind that they could never say I lacked nerve, so I used to crowd the plate closer after a pitcher had offered me a "bean" ball. That is the only way to do.
>
> I also used to come back with a lot of conversation along these lines: "You're wild enough to work with a bush league outfit. Don't think you worry me by shooting at my 'bean.' I enjoy it. Come on, I want a base on balls."
>
> If a pitcher tries to scare me away from the plate, I fight him so as to put him on the defensive, instead of letting him put me in the hole. If it become known that a hitter is "bat shy," as is indicated when he "sticks his foot in the water pail" after the pitcher aims at his head, all twirlers keep "on him." Then, if he comes up in a pinch when a hit is needed, the first thing the pitcher does is to aim one at his "bean" to scare him away. When a young player comes into the league, all the pitchers search his batting style for a weakness. As soon as one is discovered, the tip goes over the entire league, and all the twirlers aim at it. Everything is done to test and break the young player's nerve before he is admitted to fast company on an equal basis with the seasoned Big Leaguers. (Ty Cobb, *Busting 'em and Other Big League Stories*, 1914)

A Career That Fell on the Wrong Hand

Albert Leonard "Hebrew Hammer" "Flip" Rosen

Born: 1924 Died: 2015
Cleveland Indians: 1947–56
Position: Third Baseman / First Baseman
Jersey Number: 7

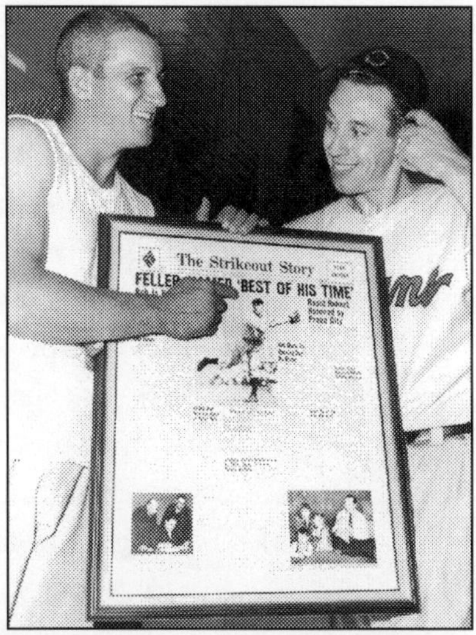

Al Rosen (left) congratulates Bob Feller for being named "the best of his time" by the Baseball Writers Association in 1951 (*The Cleveland Press* Collection, Cleveland State University, Glen Zahn, photographer)

SYMPTOMS

Al Rosen played his entire ten-year career (1947–56) with the Cleveland Indians. Rosen was a four time All-Star selection and, in 1953, the American League's Most Valuable Player. Rosen led the league that year in home runs (43), RBIs (145), and missed winning the batting average title by .001 percent, which would have given him the Triple Crown, a rare feat in major league baseball.

In the early part of the 1954 season, Rosen was asked to switch from third to first base to allow Rudy Regalado to be inserted into the lineup. Regalado was considered an up-and-coming prospect (although he never made his mark and was out of baseball a few years later). Rosen, the consummate team player agreed to make the move. On May 25, playing against the Chicago White Sox, Rosen was hit on the right hand by a ground ball and the injury began a season of pain for the Cleveland All-Star. By August, Rosen had missed fourteen games due to the broken finger (initially thought to be a sprain, but later diagnosed as a chip fracture), contusions of the chest, a bruised elbow, and bursitis of the left shoulder. Rosen was treated with a new drug—cortisone—to relieve some of the pain and allow him to stay in the lineup.

Playing through injuries was quite common during that era. The Major League Baseball Players Association wasn't formed until 1968 and without bargaining power in the 1950s, owners were prone to cut players' salaries if they had a bad season. Rosen's 1954 numbers weren't as good as his 1953 MVP season, leading to a pay cut in 1955.

The Indians went on to capture the 1954 pennant but lost in the World Series to the New York Giants. Rosen had twelve at bats during the series; he had only three hits, no home runs, and no RBIs. In the series, as was the case after the finger injury, Rosen had to bat without the use of his index finger, holding it away from the bat to avoid discomfort. Rosen's finger never healed properly, and most likely, the alteration in Rosen's swing led to other physical issues.

The Indians finished second in 1955 and 1956 and might have done better with a healthy Rosen. In 1954, Rosen's slugging percentage (total bases/at bats) was a hefty .506. In 1955, his slugging percentage dropped to .402, with a career-low .244 batting average and 21 home runs. The following year his slugging percentage rose slightly to .428, but the fans weren't on his side any more. Instead of listening to the fans' boos, Rosen decided to retire at the age of thirty-two. He became a successful stockbroker and returned to baseball twenty years later to become team president of the New York Yankees, Houston Astros, and San Francisco Giants.

PATIENT HISTORY

"A few years ago Al [Rosen] was the toast of Cleveland. . . . Today they're burning the ears of the luckless Al and it seems

rough...and much of his falling in form has been caused by injuries that he pluckily, but with questionable judgment, tries to ignore."
—*New York Times* (1956)

"I never was the same hitter after that injury and it's the reason I decided to call it a career a few years later. I couldn't stand being mediocre."
—Al Rosen

"Al Rosen seemed to burst out of his uniform. He had a thick chest. He had incredibly muscular arms. And he had a violent swing. He always seemed to be damaging the ball when [he] hit it."
—Maury Allen, sportswriter (2011)

DIAGNOSIS

Al Rosen's broken finger was a typical example of the team's injury curse. The broken finger transformed a great player who almost won the Triple Crown at age twenty-nine into an ordinary infielder who retired at thirty-two. The Tribe's magical 1954 season (with a record 111 wins) ended on a sour note and a nightmarish sweep by the Giants. The loss of Rosen in the middle of the lineup crippled the Tribe's chances in the team's best season ever.

SECOND OPINION

Rosen's bat might have helped the Tribe in the 1954 series, but even his help wouldn't have been enough. Indians' hurlers gave up two more runs per nine innings in the Giants sweep than they had over the entire regular season. While the Giants batting average in the series was a few points higher than the regular season average, the Tribe's sluggers floundered, hitting .190, seventy points below their season average. This led to a Giants ERA of 1.46 for the four-game set.

TREATMENT

Finger fractures make up ten percent of all fractures. This is not surprising, as there are fourteen bones (phalanges) in the fingers of the hand. Many treatment options are available after the bone is put back into place, including buddy taping (taping fingers together) and Coban taping (taping with elastic wrap); immobilization by the use of a cast; the use of pins or screws; and in some cases, realigning the bones after an incision and then using pins, screws, or plates.

The complications of finger fractures that are not treated or are improperly treated include the following:

Chronic deformity: The loss of function or ability to work normally because the finger is bent or twisted. (In the early years of baseball, when the game was played without gloves or with primitive gloves, "baseball finger" was a common ailment when the finger was overextended and bent directly backward.)

Chronic pain: An ailment seen most commonly in a fracture through a joint (articular fracture) and may be diagnosed as stiffness or arthritis.

Infection of the bone (osteomyelitis): A complication that usually occurs soon after a fracture because of the traumatic event.

INCIDENTAL FINDINGS

In 1973, Rosen wanted to save the struggling Cleveland franchise, which was at one of the lower points in its history. He had a deal in place with a very wealthy Clevelander, George Steinbrenner, who had agreed (in principle) to buy the franchise. The team already had called a press conference when the deal unexpectedly fell through. Shortly afterwards, Steinbrenner bought the New York Yankees and became one of the most famous and successful team owners in baseball history. Rosen and Steinbrenner turned the spotlight on New York while the Indians remained in darkness for the next two decades.

Thrown into Darkness

Herbert Jude "Herb" Score

Born: 1933 Died: 2008
Cleveland Indians:
1955–59
Position: Pitcher
Jersey Number: 27

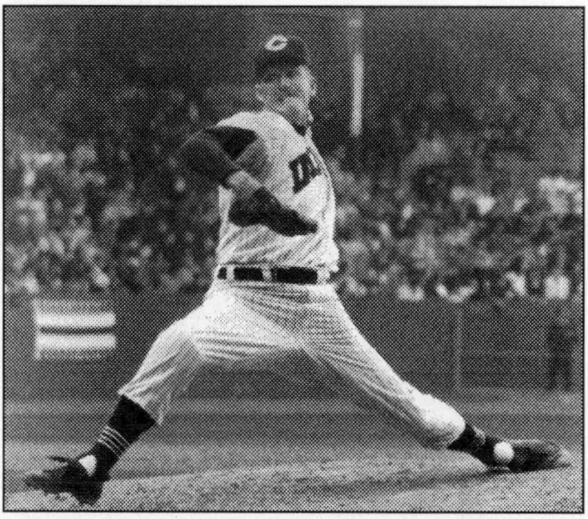

Herb Score on the mound, 1959 (*The Cleveland Press* Collection, Cleveland State University, Fred Bottomer, photographer)

SYMPTOMS

While pitching for Lake Fort Worth High School in Florida, senior Herb Score was courted by a bevy of major league scouts. Score had bouts of wildness, but when he got the ball over the plate, he was a devastating pitcher, regularly fanning batters. Score received offers from fourteen major league teams after his 1952 high school season, but chose to sign with the Indians' Indianapolis farm club for $50,000 (the figure kept escalating in media reports, reaching almost $100,000). In his first professional appearance, the Indianapolis lefty struck out four of the first five batters he faced in an exhibition game against the Cincinnati Reds.

After spending several years in the minors, Score became part of Cleveland's pitching rotation in 1955, joining future Hall of Famers Bob Feller, Bob Lemon, and Early Wynn. Score had a rookie-of-the-year record of 16–10, with 11 complete games, and a 2.85 ERA. He struck out 245 batters, a record that stood until rookie Dwight Gooden fanned 276 batters in 1984. Even with a stellar pitching staff, the 1955 Indians couldn't overtake the New York Yankees, finishing three games behind the Bronx Bombers.

Prognosticators picked the Tribe to finish fourth in 1957, since Bob Feller had retired and Lemon and Wynn were getting up in their years. In early May, the league-leading Yankees were in town for a key early season series. The Indians were only a few games out of first place and sent Herb Score to the mound. Score was viewed as the left-handed Bob Feller and with an ace like Score, the Tribe could overcome a lot of deficits and possibly contend for a pennant. An April 10, 1957, *Sporting News* profile had been released with the headline, "Will Herb Score Be the Greatest Lefthander?" He had already beaten the powerful Yankees three times in a row without much trouble.

Prior to the Yankees series, the *Cleveland Plain Dealer* was running advertisements for an article about Score that was to run in the May 11 *Saturday Evening Post,* titled "Cleveland's Left-Handed Lightning." The piece detailed many of the mishaps that had already befallen Score—being hit by a bakery truck as a three-year-old; a bout of pneumonia; an eight-week battle with rheumatic fever; a broken ankle; acute appendicitis; and a severe virus attack that had kept him out of the lineup in June 1955. The story's main focus was on his current struggle with a spastic colon caused by anxiety. His perfectionism led to pent-up frustration and self-criticism. Still, even with health problems, Score could throw his fastball by even the best American League hitters.

May 7, 1957, was a perfect day to take in a Tribe game. The weather was more summer-like than usual, reaching a daytime high of 77 degrees. A Tuesday crowd of over eighteen thousand fans came to the ballpark to see Score battle Tom "Snake" Sturdivant, who was one of the better pitchers in the league at the time. Score took the mound in the top of the first and retired leadoff hitter Hank Bauer on a ground ball. The next batter, Yankee infielder Gil McDougald, worked the count to 2–2. Score came inside with a fastball and McDougald swung. As one sportswriter described it, "I heard the crack of the bat, and the sickening thud as the blur of a baseball struck Herb Score. Score went down as if he had been shot. Blood poured from his right eye." The public address announcer, Jack Cresson, asked that any doctor in the house report to the field. Score was carried off the diamond with a severe eye injury and broken nose.

Score eventually regained his vision, but he missed the remainder of the 1957 season and part of the 1958 season. He pitched for five more years after the facial fractures, but in two years with the Indians and three years with the Chicago White Sox, his combined record was 17–26. Score retired in 1962 at the age of twenty-nine. He never blamed the injury for his pitching decline, instead saying that he had suffered a tendon tear during a cold, damp game against the Washington Senators in 1958. He also thought that the cortisone treatments he had for ten months to reduce swelling on the right side of his head might have altered his muscle tone.

In 1964, Score moved to the broadcast booth as the Cleveland Indians' television voice. He stayed in television through 1967, before joining the radio broadcast team. He remained the radio voice of the Cleveland Indians through the 1997 season—the longest career ever for an Indians play-by-play announcer. His final broadcast was game seven of the 1997 World Series, which the Indians lost to the Florida Marlins.

On October 8, 1998, Score was severely injured in a car accident in central Ohio and suffered permanent injuries from the crash. Score died on November 11, 2008, in Rocky River, Ohio.

PATIENT HISTORY

> "He would have been probably one of the greatest, if not the greatest, left-handed pitchers who ever lived."
> —Bob Feller

The gods of the diamond change like the weather,
They give us a natural and they take him forever,
And that's what they did to Herbie Score.
—Terry Cashman, "The Ballad of Herb Score"

"Once, at Indianapolis, I hit my crazy bone so hard my arm went absolutely numb. They got about ten runs in four innings off me, and I had to stay in because we didn't have anybody else available."
—Herb Score

DIAGNOSIS

Herb Score represented Cleveland Indians baseball for several generations. The late 1950s and early 1960s was a "Cleveland Camelot," when two young, good-looking stars, Score and outfielder Rocky Colavito, epitomized the future of Cleveland sports. Unfortunately, the Tribe's destiny began to unravel when Score was hit by McDougald's liner, known as "The Shot Heard around Northeast Ohio." From that point forward, Score never regained his greatness on the mound. The struggle of Herb Score and the 1960 trade of Rocky Colavito (leading to the "The Curse of Rocky Colavito") put Cleveland baseball into a dark abyss for several decades, an abyss that might have been avoided were it not for one line drive.

Herb Score will live forever in Cleveland sports lore due to the way he handled his misfortune. He moved from the mound to the broadcast booth and became the "Voice of the Tribe" during the toughest years of Indians baseball. Score certainly had his quirks and misstatements, but he was "one of us." When the Indians appeared in two World Series in the 1990s, and the bandwagon was full of Cleveland fans, everyone asked: "What did Herb think? What did Herb say? Play that audio clip from Herb again." Score fulfilled the promise of becoming a Cleveland legend; he just didn't do it with his arm.

SECOND OPINION

The 1950s were a great time to be a Tribe fan. During that decade, the team was a perennial contender, going to the World Series once, and finishing second in the American League six times. Fans showed up in droves, with attendance topping the one million mark seven times. After 1959, twenty years passed before attendance would reach that mark again.

Much of the credit for fielding competitive teams has to be given to Hank Greenberg, the Indians general manager from 1950 until 1957. However, Greenberg also caused some problems that resulted in the beginning of the Indians decline. He fired popular manager Lou Boudreau and his treatment of manager Al Lopez led to his resignation. Future Hall of Famer Luis Aparicio didn't sign with Cleveland because Greenberg wouldn't honor a handshake deal that the two had arranged.

However, Frank "Trader" Lane, the Tribe general manager from 1957 until January 1961, sent players out of Cleveland faster than lightning and left the town and the Indians reeling. Lane made sixty deals, including the unpopular trade of the well-liked Rocky Colavito. Lane also traded away Roger Maris, Norm Cash, and Early Wynn. A nucleus of Aparicio, Cash, Colavito, and Maris would have helped the Tribe win more games and draw more fans.

TREATMENT

Vehicle crashes, falls, assaults, and sports accidents frequently cause facial injuries (see medical illustration, page 296). Fractures of facial bones are associated with pain and the bruising and swelling of surrounding tissues. Initially, these fractures may cause profuse nosebleeds. Treatment is necessary to repair the normal, bony structure. Specialists, like plastic surgeons; ear, nose, and throat (ENT) surgeons; and oral surgical specialists repair the bones of the face with metal plates, screws, or wires. Bone grafting is another option to reconstruct the normal facial architecture. Surgery is usually performed within hours or days of the initial injury.

Long-term complications of facial injuries include disfigurement and disability that can cause physical scarring and emotional trauma. Such injuries can threaten eyesight and other facial functions by trapping nerves and muscles within the healing bones. The "trapdoor fracture" (a pure orbital-floor fracture, linear in form and hinged medially, which allows herniation of orbital contents through the fracture and then entraps these herniated contents) requires emergent surgery for the best outcome. Infection is another complication that must be managed. In 15–48 percent of cases, brain injuries are associated with facial trauma. In early stages, postconcussion symptoms can be overlooked while the focus of treatment is on the repair of the facial structures.

INCIDENTAL FINDINGS

Cyril Charles Slapnicka was the scout who signed Herb Score and Bob Feller to Cleveland Indians contracts. "Slap" or "Slappy," as he was called, spent most of his playing career in the minor leagues. After he hung up his spikes in late 1935, Slapnicka became the general manager for the Tribe. Earlier that year, as a scout, Slapnicka had signed the underage Bob Feller to a contract, and despite some wrangling with the league commissioner about the situation, Feller was allowed to formally sign with the club. At the time, scouts were pretty ruthless in getting players because a farm system was not fully developed and the player entry draft was decades away. Slappy also signed Bobby Avilla, Lou Boudreau, Bob Lemon, Roger Maris, and Hal Trosky. Slapnicka was in baseball from 1906 through 1960, when he retired as a scout for the Indians organization. He died in 1979 at the age of ninety-three.

Driven to the Warning Track

James Anthony "Jimmy" Piersall

Born: 1929
Cleveland Indians: 1959–61
Position: Center Fielder
Jersey Number: 37

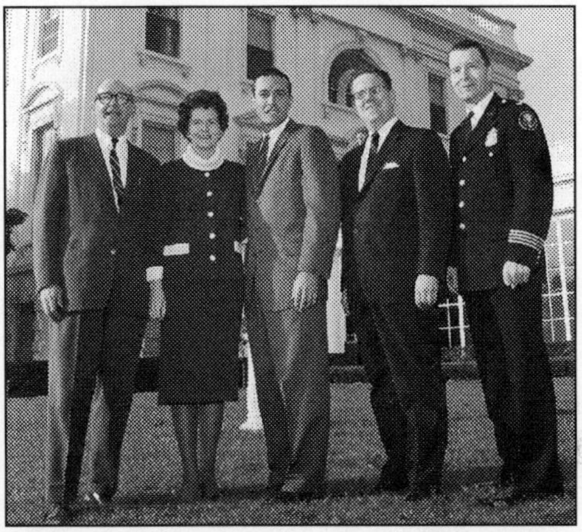

Presidential Assistants John J. McNally and David F. Powers, with Jimmy Piersall and wife Mary Piersall, 1961 (Cecil Stoughton, White House Photographs, John F. Kennedy Presidential Library and Museum, Boston)

SYMPTOMS

On December 3, 1958, the Indians traded for Boston Red Sox player Jimmy Piersall. Piersall was a superb center fielder and Casey Stengel considered him better defensively than the great Joe DiMaggio. Cleveland thought they had a team that could compete for the American League pennant the following year, and in addition to Piersall, they had acquired the scrappy Billy Martin. Martin knew Piersall—he had goaded Martin, then a Yankee, into a brawl during the 1952 season. By the time Piersall arrived in Cleveland, he had a reputation as unstable and for doing outlandish things, including "oinking" at Satchel Paige during a game. Near the end of his rookie season, Boston sent him to the minors. Shortly after, Piersall ended up in the Westborough (MA) State Hospital for psychiatric treatment, which included electroshock therapy.

In 1957, Piersall's struggles reached the big screen. Based on his autobiography of the same name, the film *Fear Strikes Out* featured

Anthony Perkins as Piersall and Karl Malden starring as the ballplayer's father. While today's tell-all stories might be run of the mill, Piersall's admissions about his bipolar disorder were stunning in an era when most Americans were unaware of the many faces of mental illness. The movie did more than document Piersall's life in and out of baseball. Fans used the information to heckle Piersall about his illness, which exacerbated the situation.

With the Indians, Piersall continued to make waves. On one occasion he pulled a squirt gun from his pocket and sprayed home plate so the umpire could get a better view of the strike zone. He had to be rescued by teammates after he challenged fans in the Yankee Stadium bleachers to a fight. In June 1960, Piersall threw a baseball and an orange at Comiskey Park's exploding scoreboard. Later that month, after the Yankees pitcher Jim Coates threw a pitch at Piersall for supposedly timing his warm-up pitches, Piersall responded by throwing a bat at Coates. Piersall had run-ins with umpires and teammates, and while he had periods of relative calm, his behavior did not always fit within the lines.

As Cleveland challenged for the pennant in 1959, Piersall didn't provide the needed offense, batting only .233 and playing in only 100 games. Used many times as a pinch hitter, he chose to sit in the bullpen instead of the dugout. Martin didn't help much either, batting only .260, and he was traded to Cincinnati a year later. Piersall's batting prowess returned in 1960 and 1961 when he hit .282 and .322 respectively. He also won his second Gold Glove as a Tribe outfielder in 1961, but the Tribe didn't win the top spot in the American League and traded Piersall to the Washington Senators for four players, including pitcher Dick Donavan.

PATIENT HISTORY

"Probably the best thing that ever happened to me was going nuts. It brought people out to the ballpark to get a look at me, and they came to places I was invited to speak."
—Jimmy Piersall

"[H]e had the umpires so worked up that they'd never give us a break."
—Frank Lane, Cleveland Indians general manager

"Piersall's greatest contribution to baseball lay in his insistence that the game should be fun to play. He consistently displayed a keen wit, a questionable sense of humor and a zany joie de vivre that some fans loved."
—Albert Kilchesty, baseball historian

"[N]o one seems sure how the Martians would react to Jimmy Piersall."
—Chuck Heaton, Cleveland sportswriter

DIAGNOSIS

Jimmy Piersall gave Cleveland fans an interesting three years from 1959 to 1961. During what was already a turbulent time for the Tribe, things became more interesting with Piersall's antics. General Manager Frank "Trader" Lane was in the process of dismantling the team, which led to a steady decline for the once promising Indians. Not knowing what might happen when Piersall took the field probably distracted fans from the fact that the Tribe was not a perennial contender anymore. The Indians' outfielder played the game in his own way and when he was unburdened by his demons, he showed joy and skill that the fans loved. After his father died of an apparent heart attack in September 1961, Piersall ended up in a fight with two fans who had bolted onto the field in Yankee Stadium. The event was probably the last one Cleveland management could endure; Piersall was traded less than a month later.

SECOND OPINION

After the Piersall trade, the Tribe dropped from first in batting average in 1961 (.275) to last in 1962 (.245). Dick Donovan had a career year in 1962, going 20–10, but the Indians' pitching staff posted the same ERA as they had in 1961. Donovan never had a winning season afterward and retired in 1965 after pitching a little over twenty-two innings that year with a record of 1–3. The other three players that came to Cleveland in the deal were primarily backups.

TREATMENT

Bipolar disorder is also known as manic-depressive disorder. A person with this disorder exhibits abnormally elevated moods or energy levels followed by abnormally depressed states that interfere with normal functioning. Genetic factors can contribute greatly to the development of the disorder, but environmental factors can also play a role. The onset of bipolar symptoms typically occurs early in life, between the midteenage years and early twenties. While it is difficult to ascertain an exact estimate because of misdiagnosis and the social stigma associated with the disorder, between 1–1.5 percent of the population have this disorder.

The symptoms of the manic phase may include changes in sleep patterns (very little deep sleep per night), rapid speech, and a short attention span. In the depressive stage, an individual may feel sadness, guilt, anger, isolation, or hopelessness, and may also exhibit periods of fatigue, apathy, and irritability. Individuals with bipolar disorder have a high suicide rate (33 percent of those diagnosed with bipolar disorder attempt suicide). The long-standing treatment is lithium, but anticonvulsants like Depakote and Tegretol, in combination, are now used for difficult cases.

INCIDENTAL FINDINGS

Prior to Paramount's 1957 release of *Fear Strikes Out: The Jimmy Piersall Story*, CBS television produced an hour-long drama starring actor Tab Hunter based on the book. The big screen version garnered a lot of support, though some sportswriters were skeptical of mental illness in a masculine sport like baseball. The *New York Times*' review of the film attributed Piersall's problems to neurasthenia, nervous exhaustion. While mental illness was not well understood in the 1950s, even as early as 1888, the general public considered symptoms of neurasthenia "largely of a subjective character, and to one who does not suffer them, appear trifling and unreal." Still, the *New York Times*' review did note, "The weight of paternal ambition is the central factor in this film. And it is felt by the nerve-racked observer to the point where it is recognizable that the young man [Piersall] must go mad" (March 21, 1957).

No Hard and Fastball Rules

Samuel Edward "Sudden Sam" McDowell

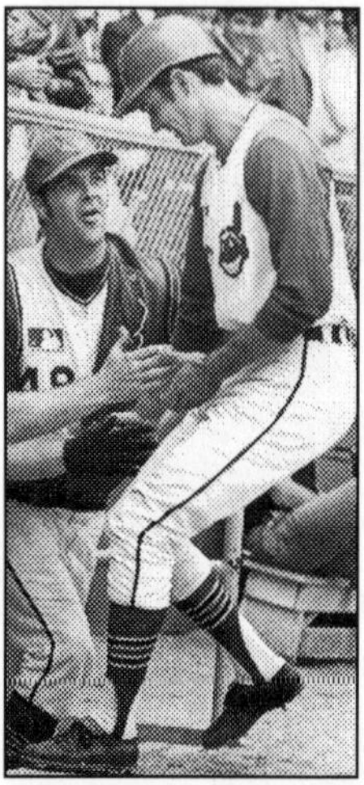

Born: 1942
Cleveland Indians: 1961–71
Position: Pitcher
Jersey Number: 48

Sam McDowell congratulates Vern Fuller after a home run, 1969 (*The Cleveland Press Collection*, Cleveland State University, Paul Tepley, photographer)

SYMPTOMS

As a seventeen-year-old high schooler, Sam McDowell struck out 152 batters in 63 innings and did not allow an earned run. In his Little League, sandlot, and scholastic careers he recorded forty no-hitters. To say that major league teams wanted to sign him to a contract in 1960 is closer to a lie than an understatement. McDowell was six foot five, around 225 pounds, and possessed a fastball that was compared to the fireballs of Bob Feller and Sandy Koufax.

Followed by scouts for over two years, McDowell had pitched two no-hitters and a one-hitter in the 1959 Colt World Series in Los Angeles. Competition was stern for the kid from Pittsburgh's Central Catholic High, but the Indians won the bidding war by offering the teenager a $75,000 signing bonus.

In 1959, the Indians had an 89–65 record, good for second place—five games behind the White Sox. Though McDowell would need some time in the minors, the Indians seemed to be building for the future. All-Star Rocky Colavito had blasted out 42 home runs and had 111 RBIs in 1959; maybe Herb Score could return. Impetuous Frank "Trader" Lane couldn't see the team's promise and traded the popular Colavito to Detroit, beginning what some have termed "The Curse of Rocky Colavito"—a downward spiral for Indians' fans.

After a brief appearance in 1961, McDowell came up for good in 1962. He was a Tribe starter until 1971 and recorded 122 wins. He was a six-time All-Star selection, leading the American League in ERA and strikeouts in 1965, strikeouts and shutouts in 1966, and strikeouts again in 1968. In 1970, he was named Pitcher of the Year by *Sporting News* after winning twenty games for the only time in his career. During his major league tenure, he averaged almost nine strikeouts per outing. His record dropped to 13–17 in 1971 and Sudden Sam was traded to San Francisco for Gaylord Perry and shortstop Frank Duffy. McDowell's contract was eventually purchased by the Yankees and he finished his career with the Pittsburgh Pirates.

McDowell never reached his full potential, due in part to what Indians sportscaster Bob Neal called a million-dollar arm with a ten-cent head. Everyone marveled at his talent but he was always more of a thrower than a pitcher. He loved challenges, but once he'd overcome them he'd be more inclined to throw other pitches to lesser hitters for variety's sake, if nothing else. McDowell claimed he had low self-esteem in his early years in the Big Leagues and found an ally in the bottle. If McDowell had worked harder and gotten treatment, his record could have mirrored the best pitchers in major league history.

PATIENT HISTORY

> "I had all the traits [of an alcoholic]: Show off. You're the big shot. Mr. Cool. Defiant of authority. Difficulty finishing anything. A loner."
>
> —Sam McDowell

"Although he was a great pitcher, we called him Sad Sam McDowell because he didn't accomplish as much with the wonderful talent he had as he should have."
—Bill Kinnamon, major league umpire

"There are things you can do when you have talent that are colorful. If you do them without talent, they're bush. Sam has talent."
—Gabe Paul, Cleveland general manager

"Sudden makes it like it used to be when we were kids. You know he's gonna challenge you.... As a matter of fact, I think he'd be tougher if he had less ability. Sudden just has too much stuff!"
—Reggie Jackson, Hall of Famer

DIAGNOSIS

Sam McDowell was constantly compared to the best pitchers of all time, including Bob Feller and Sandy Koufax. A part of the equation was always missing, however, and Sudden Sam exited baseball at a relatively young age. Was it his attitude? Was it coaching? Was low self-esteem to blame for Sam's alcoholism? Although McDowell was part of many dreadful Indians' teams (one above-500 season), when McDowell was on the mound, fans saw glimpses of greatness.

In an era before free agency, McDowell was never able to play for a contender. His story might have turned out much differently if he played for the Yankees in his prime. Cleveland management had to hold on to its stars, especially when the teams surrounding those stars weren't capable of producing the kind of statistics that could lead to the postseason. During the McDowell era, fans went to August and September games hoping the Tribe could derail others team's pennant dreams.

SECOND OPINION

If pitching, defense, and timely hitting led to pennants, the 1964–70 Indians were on a long road to nowhere. In the ten-team American League, the Tribe booted balls around Cleveland Stadium regularly. The best they finished during the span was fifth in errors committed. They were ninth twice and led the league in errors committed in 1965.

Tribe hitting wasn't much better. The best year was in 1965, when the Indians finished third in the league in batting average. Eliminating that year, the Tribe averaged around seventh each year.

Going to the mound knowing run production was not forthcoming and the defense wasn't sound had to put extra pressure on the Tribe staff. McDowell pitched with several sound hurlers including Luis Tiant, Sonny Siebert, and at times, Steve Hargan. Without support, odds weren't in their favor.

TREATMENT

About fourteen million Americans suffer from alcoholism. Alcoholics and alcohol abusers are recurrently and persistently beset with an urge to drink, an urge that is compelling enough for them to continue to drink despite the fact that because of their drinking they sustain substantial damage to their health and personal or business affairs.

Alcoholism has long-term effects, including increased tolerance of and dependence on alcohol. Physical symptoms include liver inflammation or cirrhosis, pancreatitis, dementia, heart disease, and nutritional deficiencies. Social problems vary from person to person, but may include child abuse, domestic violence, burglary, and assault. Alcoholism can also lead to loss of employment, financial/legal problems, and marital conflict or divorce.

There are many environmental factors that lead to the development of alcoholism, but genetics often play a significant role. Treatment involves a multifaceted approach, which includes life training, social support, and attendance at self-help groups. The first step is often a detoxification or abrupt stoppage of alcohol consumption. Drugs such as benzodiazepines may be necessary during this period.

In the sixties, the coolness of alcohol, epitomized by the three-martini lunch, pervaded society and was spurred on by advertisers. More recently, sports franchises have addressed the problem and have provided more avenues for help. In many ways, players in the sixties were expected to party hard and play hard as well.

INCIDENTAL FINDINGS

When baseball became professionalized in the late 1800s, players did not always have pristine characters. In fact, the public thought baseball had its share of hooligans, gamblers, and drunks. Baseball needed an image change to gain popularity. Connie Mack, who spent seventy-one years in baseball and is known as its grand old gentleman, laid it on the line to ballplayers.

> There has been a great change in baseball during the past fifteen years. This has been due in a great measure to the class of men who are now making up baseball teams. In former years, players did not receive very high salaries, and naturally we did not get the class of players whom we are getting today, as the salaries are now very high, and we have in our profession, I might say fully fifty per cent, of college players. The balance of our players with a very few exceptions, are all well-educated men. Alcoholism is practically eliminated from baseball. For instance, I have twenty-five players. Of that number, fifteen don't know the taste of liquors. The few remaining, may, possibly, after a game of ball, take a glass of beer. They do not make a practice of this. Neither do we restrict them from doing so if they desire. They know that we do not approve of their drinking, and the positions

that they hold, and the salary that they receive keep them from any such thought as becoming accustomed to drink. I often get into an argument caused by remarks that such and such a player had been seen taking a glass of beer. There is no class of professional men that is watched so closely as the baseball players. If seen taking a drink, a rumor is immediately started that the player was seen drunk last night. This travels very swiftly and is a great injustice to the player, who would not under any circumstances take the second drink. I have had so many arguments that I usually put the matter in this way: Take twenty-five from the baseball profession, and the same number from any bank or brokerage house, and you will find that the percentage using intoxicating liquors is far greater with the latter. I actually believe that in five years from this date at least ninety per cent of the players will be strictly temperate. (Connie Mack, "Baseball Players Must Be Sober," *Scientific Temperance Journal*, 1909)

An Unfortunate New York Run-In

Leon Lamar "Daddy Wags" Wagner

Cleveland Indians: 1964–67
Born: 1934 Died: 2004
Position: Left Fielder
Jersey Number: 27

Larry Leslie "Brownie" Brown

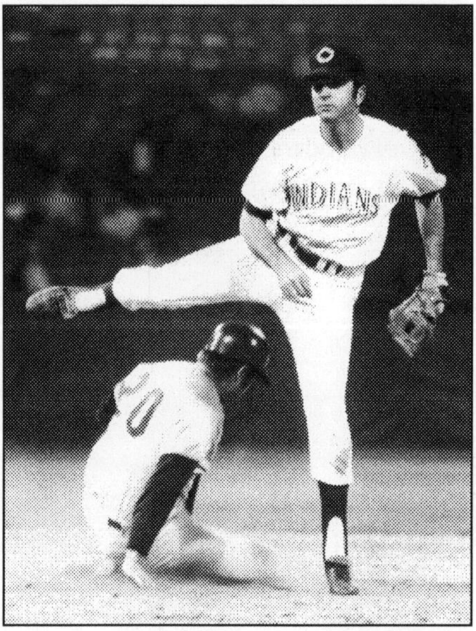

Born: 1940
Cleveland Indians: 1963–71
Position: Shortstop
Jersey Number: 16

Cleveland shortstop, Larry Brown eludes a sliding runner, 1970 (*The Cleveland Press* Collection, Cleveland State University, Paul Tepley, photographer)

SYMPTOMS

After an above-500 finish in 1965, Cleveland fans hoped for further improvement in 1966. Leon "Daddy Wags" Wagner, a 1963 acquisition from the California Angels (Skylark Records released a single by Wendy Cole and the Twilighters called "The Wiggle Wiggle" named after the slugger's idiosyncrasies at the plate) had come off a season where he batted .294, with 28 home runs and 79 RBIs. Cleveland rooters hoped Wagner could continue to provide home-run power in the Cleveland lineup. After all, his familiar saying was "Have no fear. Daddy Wags is here!"

Larry Brown was a light-hitting but defensively talented middle infielder for the Tribe from 1963–71. Brownie, as he was called, was signed in 1958 out of Lake Worth High School in Florida, where he was an All-Conference player. The school had also produced Cleveland pitcher Herb Score (see page 23). Brown would never be confused with Daddy Wags at the plate, and their paths crossed in an unfortunate way for the Tribe.

May 4, 1966, was an unusually warm day in New York City, with the temperature reaching a high of 86 degrees. The Indians sent Sonny Siebert to the mound against Yankee Mel Stottlemyre in the afternoon contest. The game turned into a pitcher's duel, eventually won 2–1 by the Indians.

With two out in the fourth inning, Yankee great Roger Maris stepped to the plate. Siebert hadn't allowed a hit up to that point. Maris lifted a soft fly ball up the left field line. Brown rushed toward the ball from shortstop and Wagner ran from left field. The ball was dropping quickly and both players aimed to catch it. Wagner and Brown collided; a sickening crack of their heads could be heard throughout the ballpark. Both players crumbled to the ground. Brown had swallowed his tongue, and Indian trainer Wally Bock got it loose or Brown might have died on the spot. Brown was rushed to a nearby hospital for further treatment.

Brown suffered multiple fractures of the skull and fractures of the nose and cheek. "Cheeky," a Wagner nickname due to the high cheek bones inherited from his Choctaw ancestors, broke his nose and suffered facial lacerations.

Brown awoke three days later and wasn't allowed to get out of bed for over ten days. The Tribe announced that Brown's season was over. He stayed in the hospital a total of eighteen days. In the end, Brown would return after forty-three days, but his batting average suffered, dropping from .262 to .229. Wagner continued to play, but his power numbers dropped and continued to do so for the next two years. He was traded in June 1968 to the Chicago White Sox.

At the time of the collision, the Tribe was 13–1 and in first place. The streaky Chico Salmon replaced Brown during his recuperation. Salmon actually hit well, but his fielding was not as good as Brown's. The unexpected accident impacted the Tribe's power numbers, too. By season's end, the Tribe had fired manager Birdie Tebbetts and finished at 81–81.

Wagner's postbaseball life was anything but happy. He tried his hand at running a clothing store, but the effort failed. He was ambushed and shot by two intruders in 1972. The last years of his life were spent homeless in the Crenshaw section of Los Angeles. Larry Brown ended up in Florida after his baseball career was over.

PATIENT HISTORY

> "As kids, we grew-up poor, but I learned to hit using a broomstick and a golf ball. When I finally got a bat, it was like a big club. When I saw the baseball coming at me, it looked like a basketball being thrown at me."
> —Leon Wagner

> "[N]othing against Cleveland—but I'd rather have been traded somewhere in the United States."
> —Leon Wagner, after the 1963 trade from the Angels to Cleveland

> "I could hardly recognize him. If the doctors hadn't told me that was Larry's bed, I wouldn't have recognized him. I was shocked when I saw him."
> —Helen Brown, Larry's wife

DIAGNOSIS

Any Cleveland sports fan who was alive in the 1960s remembers the collision between Daddy Wags and Brownie. The Tribe made national news, if for all the wrong reasons. Games came to most households via radio then and fans read the morning newspapers to find out about the Tribe. The collision was the lead story on page one of the *Plain Dealer*, which included a picture of the two players lying unconscious on the field.

Perhaps with a bit of hyperbole, the *Plain Dealer* reported that the Indians' pennant hopes had taken a severe blow, but fans always wanted to believe. Still, teams win championships, not individuals. Ultimately, though, the collision impacted two starters and the entire season.

SECOND OPINION

The Indians of 1966 weren't fleet of foot. The team was dead last in the league in doubles and triples. Rocky Colavito had returned the previous year with a stellar season, driving in 108 runs to lead the league. Perhaps the curse was finally being lifted.

The Tribe ranked third in the American League in pitching in 1966. The collision between Wagner and Brown wasn't the only factor in the team's decline after a great start. Colavito showed his age and drove in 36 fewer runs than the previous year. The Tribe's starting lineup changed frequently as players sat out with minor injuries. Third baseman Max Alvis started and finished the most games, 157 started and 152 finished. Without reliable power hitters, the team couldn't score enough runs and hit into too many double plays.

TREATMENT

In 1966, interest in skull fractures revolved around injuries in automobile accidents, especially with the increased use of safety glass. Seat belt laws wouldn't come into effect until decades later.

A skull fracture is a break in one or more of the bones of the cranial vault. The direct impact that causes the fracture may cause damage to the blood vessels or to the brain. The injury can cause a brain bleed or a concussion; however, some uncomplicated skull fractures occur without physical or neurologic damage. A skull fracture warrants a complete neurologic and radiologic exam to determine management and prognosis of the injury.

When Wagner and Brown collided, techniques like CAT scans were not prevalent, although symptoms of a fracture in Brown were quite evident—bleeding from the wound caused by the trauma near the location of the trauma, or around the eyes, ears, and nose; bruising around the trauma area, under the eyes, or behind the ears; pain at the site of the trauma; swelling at the injured area; and redness or warmth at the trauma site.

INCIDENTAL FINDINGS

The Glasgow Coma Scale (GCS) has been the gold standard of neurologic assessment for trauma patients since its development in the early 1970s. The scale measures eye, verbal, and motor responses. Scores of less than eight indicate a severe head injury; scores of nine to twelve indicate a moderate head injury; and scores of thirteen to fifteen indicate a mild head injury. While not available at the time of the Wagner-Brown collision, from the media reports it is quite clear that Brown's score would have been considered severe.

Driven Out of the Game

Anthony Darrin "Tony" Horton

Born: 1944
Cleveland Indians:
1967–70
Position: First
Baseman / Left Fielder
Jersey Number: 11

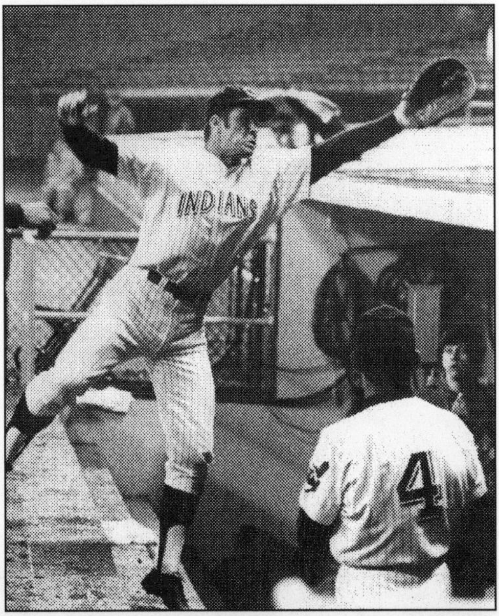

Tony Horton strains to catch a foul ball, 1970 (*The Cleveland Press* Collection, Cleveland State University, Paul Tepley, photographer)

SYMPTOMS

After an 81–81 season in 1966, the Tribe was 23–22 on June 15, 1967. The Boston Red Sox were 24–22 at the time and needed pitching to make a run at the American League pennant. Indians General Manager Gabe Paul wanted a slugger who could help the team for many seasons, and sent right-hander Gary "Ding-Dong" Bell to Boston for first baseman and outfielder Tony Horton and utility player Don Demeter. Horton was the key player in the deal for the Tribe.

A budding young star, Horton was from Southern California, stood over six foot tall, and weighed 210 pounds. The first baseman was a high-strung perfectionist, but as Ted Williams noted, Horton had a natural swing that couldn't be easily taught. When Horton heard of the trade, he was thankful to get a chance to show what he could do, since his playing time in Boston was limited. In 106 games with Cleveland in 1967, Horton batted .281, with 10 home runs and 44 RBIs. The following year he slugged out 14 home runs and drove in 59 runs. His best year was 1969, when the twenty-four-year-old Horton hit 27 home runs and had 93 RBIs. Tribe fans thought they had found the next Rocky Colavito. Unfortunately, 1970 would be Horton's last year in Cleveland and in baseball.

The beginning of 1970 found Horton in a salary dispute with Cleveland general manager and field manager Alvin Dark. Horton felt his 1969 numbers afforded him a pay increase. Dark felt differently, and Horton didn't report to spring training. The conflict played out in the local papers and there were reports that Horton's teammates weren't on his side. The Cleveland slugger wanted upwards of $65,000, almost $25,000 more than the Tribe was offering. Eventually, Horton got $50,000, but the negotiations had made Horton a villain to some fans, which was a blow to Horton's fragile psyche.

Boos started early for Horton in mid-May when he was on a 6–41 hitting slump. By June and July, Horton hit better; he led the team in RBIs and was second in home runs. The holdout for more money, however, had a lingering effect and fans heckled him regularly.

Perhaps the start of Horton's final demise can be traced to a July 24 game against the Yankees in New York. Horton came to bat against Steve Hamilton, who was known to throw the "folly floater," a pitch released high into the air that drifted to the plate in a very slow manner. Horton fouled off the first floater. On the second floater, Horton took a monstrous swing and fouled the ball behind the plate, where Thurmon Munson caught it for an out. Horton walked back to the dugout, dropped to his knees, and crawled down the steps.

The following week Horton was late for a game and was fined. Then he went into a sustained batting slump and the fans let him know they disapproved in no uncertain terms. Letters to the city's sports pages lambasted Horton. In late August, Horton was pulled from the second game of a doubleheader due to a groin injury.

Finally, on September 9, the Indians' team doctor confirmed that Horton was out for the remainder of the season, due to physical exhaustion. In fact, Horton was hospitalized due to emotional problems; his playing days were over. Years later, it was reported that Horton had tried to commit suicide. Instead of ten more years of consistent and perhaps improving power numbers, the Indians were without a first baseman and Tony Horton was advised not to talk about his baseball career again.

PATIENT HISTORY

"I don't think I ever knew a more intense player than Tony Horton."
—Gabe Paul, Cleveland Indians president

"Tony was a stud. He was as good a hitter as I ever saw."
—Craig Nettles, Cleveland Indians third baseman

"I just can't understand what I'm doing wrong. I know I should relax and I tell myself to relax every time I go to the plate. But I don't. I can't, but don't ask me why."
—Tony Horton, July 1970

"[B]aseball is no longer a part of my life and that's the way I want it."
—Tony Horton, July 1973

DIAGNOSIS

The Indians finally got something right in the late 1960s when they traded a serviceable starting pitcher for a budding star. By most accounts, Tony Horton should have played another decade while putting up numbers like his 1969 season, yet his career was abruptly ended by mental illness. The series of events that contributed to his breakdown were unfortunate and were perhaps avoidable. The Indians and Alvin Dark were determined to low ball Horton despite his powerful breakout season in 1969; he was rewarded with a paltry $1,000 raise. The Indians' ownership should never have allowed the manager to negotiate player contracts. Dark was a power-hungry, egotistical dictator and he turned on the young star and manipulated the media into portraying Horton as greedy.

The Tribe compounded the problem by overpaying for Ken Harrelson (see page 53) to pressure Horton into signing. Ironically, Horton inked his contract the day before Harrelson broke his ankle. After a slow start on the field, the fans were bitter about bad baseball, front office mismanagement, and a lack of capital. Dark shifted the blame to the young slugger and the fans vented their anger at the first baseman. Horton broke down under the weight of boos and barbs.

SECOND OPINION

Alvin Dark was a manager who had a very narrow perspective on players and their needs. His views about African American and Latino ballplayers drew criticism. During his San Francisco managing career he forbade players from speaking in Spanish and from playing Latin music in the clubhouse. Perhaps Dark felt that chiding Horton would inspire the first baseman to play better.

The premature loss of Horton hurt the Indians' offense. However, other Alvin Dark trades damaged the team even more. Dark traded away Luis Tiant, Stan Williams, Max Alvis, and Duke Sims. Dark was impetuous and had unlimited authority, a combination that did not work in the Tribe's favor. In 1968, the Tribe staff had the best ERA in the league. Two years later, their ERA was ninth out of twelve teams.

TREATMENT

Clinical depression or major depressive disorder is a mental disorder characterized by low mood, low self-esteem, loss of interest and pleasure, and feelings of helplessness and hopelessness. People with this disorder often withdraw from social situations and may have thoughts of suicide. For a diagnosis of clinical depression, five or more of the following symptoms must occur over a two-week period, most of the day, nearly every day. At least one of the symptoms must be either a depressed mood or a loss of interest or pleasure. Signs and symptoms may include:

- Depressed mood, such as feeling sad, empty or tearful (in children and teens, depressed mood can appear as constant irritability)
- Significantly reduced interest or feeling no pleasure in all or most activities
- Significant weight loss when not dieting, weight gain, or decrease or increase in appetite (in children, failure to gain weight as expected)
- Insomnia or increased desire to sleep
- Either restlessness or slowed behavior that can be observed by others
- Fatigue or loss of energy
- Feelings of worthlessness, or excessive or inappropriate guilt
- Trouble making decisions, or trouble thinking or concentrating
- Recurrent thoughts of death or suicide, or a suicide attempt

Current biological theories into the nature of depression focus on serotonin, norepinephrine, and dopamine, which are naturally occurring chemicals in the brain that assist communication between brain cells. Treatment for clinical depression may include psychotherapy, medication, and electroconvulsive therapy (ECT).

Medications target these naturally occurring chemicals. There have been great advances in the number and type of drugs available to help treat the disorder. Serotonin reuptake inhibitors are currently the most common, including Paxel, Prozac, Zoloft, and Celexa. ECT, a procedure where a patient's brain is pulsed with electricity to induce a seizure, is reserved for the most refractory or significant cases. The median duration of a depressive episode is twenty-three months, with the highest rate of recovery in the first three months.

INCIDENTAL FINDINGS

Tony Horton's attempted suicide had to have had a chilling effect on Gabe Paul. In 1940, a younger Paul was the travelling secretary for the Cincinnati Reds. The backup catcher was Willard Herschberger, who was in his third year with the team. During an August trip to Boston to play the Bees, Herschberger saw action in a Friday double-header, but went hitless in five at bats.

The following day, Herschberger didn't show up at the ballpark for an afternoon game. Paul called the hotel and talked with the catcher, who said he was sick and couldn't play, but would be right over. After Herschberger failed to show up, Daniel Cohen, a close friend of Herschberger's who was in Boston with the team, went to the hotel. The door was locked and Herschberger did not answer; Cohen was let in by the hotel staff. Tragically, Herschberger was found in the bathroom in a pool of blood; he had slit his throat with a razor. Paul had been the last person to talk with the catcher.

Teammates later indicated that Herschberger was depressed over his failure to consistently play well. The Reds went on to win the 1940 World Series. Afterwards, the team voted to give a full share of the World Series earnings to Herschberger's mother, Maude. Mrs. Herschberger had lost both her husband and her son to suicide.

All That Glitters Isn't Golden

Kenneth Smith "The Hawk" Harrelson

Born: 1941
Cleveland Indians: 1969–71
Position: First Baseman / Right Fielder
Jersey Number: 40

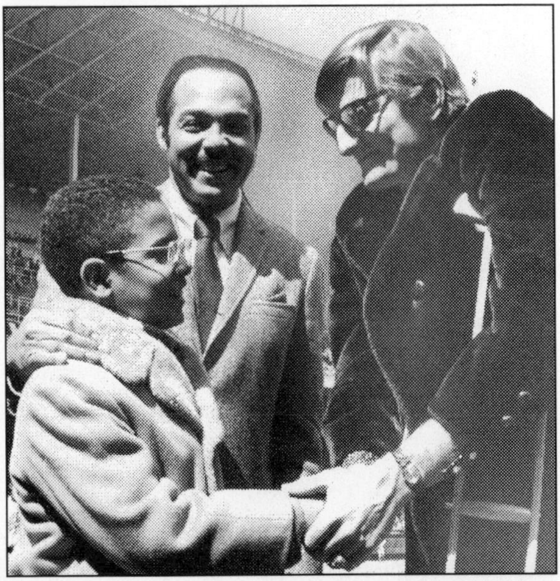

"Hawk" Harrelson, on crutches, greets Mayor Carl B. Stokes and his son on Opening Day, 1970 (*The Cleveland Press* Collection, Cleveland State University, Bernie Noble, photographer)

SYMPTOMS

Ken Harrelson came to baseball at the right time. He was "far-out" during the heyday of the 1968–73 television series *The Mod Squad*, a drama that featured three hip youths who avoided jail by becoming undercover Los Angeles cops. Harrelson's flamboyant style and outspoken character made him a favorite of the rebellious generation. Sporting a Beatle-style haircut, love beads, Nehru jackets, and dark glasses, "The Hawk" was the opposite of many of his crew-cut managers and teammates.

As a member of the Kansas City Athletics, he once reportedly called the team's owner Charles Finley "a menace to baseball" after Finley fired the team's manager, Alvin Dark. Finley released the outfielder outright and Harrelson ended up with the Boston Red Sox, signing a very large contract for the era of $75,000. He helped the Red Sox win the pennant in 1967 and was an All-Star and the *Sporting News'* Player of the Year in 1968, blasting out 35 home runs and amassing 109 RBIs.

Harrelson was a fierce competitor in many ways, probably because he had a difficult childhood. His parents were divorced and his mother raised him and his sister on a meager income. An early lesson in business came when he was being recruited to play sports for a Georgia high school. A booster who owned a local gas company offered to pay Harrelson forty dollars a week to paint gas tanks. Also included were a gas heater and free gas, which was a huge savings for the low income family.

Harrelson was not one to shy away from headlines. During a 1964 winter league baseball game in Venezuela, Harrelson was suspended fifteen days and fined $445 for exchanging punches with an umpire. During his Boston career cherry bombs were tossed at him from Tiger Stadium's upper deck and he refused to go back out onto the field. He was not timid about arguing with umpires and was ejected for his opinions on many occasions.

On April 19, 1969, the Red Sox shocked Harrelson by trading him to the Cleveland Indians, along with Juan Pizarro and Dick Ellsworth, in exchange for Sonny Siebert, Joe Azcue, and Vincente Romo. Harrelson briefly retired in protest and said he would become a pro golfer. Following conversations with Major League Baseball Commissioner Bowie Kuhn and a contract adjustment, Harrelson reported to Cleveland and slugged 27 home runs and had 84 RBIs for the Indians.

A box-office draw, Harrelson seemed primed for the 1970 season; that outlook changed in spring training. As the *Plain Dealer* reported, "[T]he optimism that had been growing was replaced with gloom and despondency. Ken (The Hawk) Harrelson, who was expected to be the team's slugging and inspirational leader, suffered a fracture of the fibula bone in the right leg" (March 20, 1970). After further examination the injury appeared even worse than originally thought. The Hawk had also suffered torn ligaments, tendon damage, and a dislocation to his right ankle. Harrelson ended up only playing in 17 games near the end of the 1970 season. He came back in 1971 and appeared in 52 games, hitting only .199, with 5 home runs. Deciding that he did indeed want to pursue a professional golf career, he retired from baseball in early June 1971. His golf career never materialized and he ended up in the broadcast booth for the Chicago White Sox. He has held that position for over twenty years; he has been voted Illinois Sportscaster of the Year twice, and has won five Emmy Awards.

PATIENT HISTORY

> "There's no way I ever considered Ken Harrelson, baseball player, to be stupid. I mean, anybody who gets paid $100,000 for hitting .221 must be very, very smart."
> —Russell Schneider, Cleveland sportswriter

> "I feel that all my life baseball has been my worst game and golf has been my best game, so why not try what you're best at?"
> —Ken Harrelson, 1971

> "As long as Harrelson hits, he can wear his hair as long as he likes."
> — Dick O'Connell, Boston general manager

DIAGNOSIS

The Cleveland Indians wanted Ken Harrelson's flamboyant style as much as the home runs he hit. The Hawk was acquired as much to keep fans interested in his persona off the field, as well as his play on the field. Unfortunately, the Tribe gave up three good players, including Sonny Siebert, an especially strong starting pitcher, to acquire Harrelson. At the time of the trade, the Indians' front office might have overrated Harrelson's talent. By 1971, the team was hindered by the lopsided trade because Harrelson failed to make a lasting impact. His one full season in Boston was definitely a career year. The Hawk acquisition followed a trend at the time—trading away the future for a quick fix. The ride Harrelson took the Indians' fans on in 1969 was all too brief, making him one of the fastest flameouts in Tribe history.

SECOND OPINION

The Tribe's management didn't help the club by acquiring Harrelson. In 1968, the year prior to the Hawk's arrival, the club drew almost 858,000 fans, had the best ERA in the league, and was third best in wins. In the Hawk's first year, the Tribe drew about 620,000 fans, were tenth in ERA, and dead last in wins. Harrelson added power to a team that managed 75 home runs in 1968, but the team's batting average only went up by .03 percent in 1969. At times, not making a trade is the best trade. The Hawk didn't fly so well on the shores of Lake Erie.

TREATMENT

Ankle fractures, accounting for about 15–25 percent of all injuries sustained by athletes, are categorized into many types, varying in severity and healing time. An X-ray or MRI scan is usually needed to discover the fracture.

Types of ankle fractures include:

- Avulsion Fracture (attached ligament or tendon pulls off a piece of the bone)
- Closed fracture (bone doesn't break the skin)
- Open fracture (bone breaks the skin, which causes an increased risk of infection)
- Displaced fracture (bones are moved from their normal position)

- Nondisplaced fracture (bones are not moved significantly from their normal position)
- Comminuted fracture (bone breaks into three or more pieces)
- Greenstick—bone is bent (bone does not break completely or breaks only on one side; occurs mainly in children)
- Growth plate fracture (bone breaks in area of soft growth cartilage where bone is still growing; this fracture only occurs in children)
- Buckle fracture (bone buckles in against the opposite side of the bone; this fracture only occurs in children)
- Stress fracture (small crack in the bone usually from overuse; also called microfracture)

Typical treatment requires immobilization with a cast or boot if the fracture is adequately aligned. Otherwise, surgery is required if the X-ray shows the need for alignment. When the ankle joint is not aligned correctly, or will not stay aligned correctly with a cast, the uneven surface of the joint will lead to arthritis and long-term problems with mobility.

INCIDENTAL FINDINGS

Ken Harrelson is credited with wearing batting gloves for the first time in a major league game in 1964. Prior to a Kansas City Athletics game against the Yankees, Harrelson had played several rounds of golf and developed blisters on his hands. To minimize the pain while batting Harrelson wore golf gloves. Players on both teams thought it was simply another Hawk eccentricity. However, after Harrelson had a terrific night at the plate, including slugging two home runs, players showed up to subsequent games with golf gloves, too. A trend had begun.

The Hawk was unsuccessful as a professional golfer. He ended up playing in nine pro tournaments and only made the cut once. His first start was in August 1971 when he played at the Little American Golf Classic, a PGA satellite event, at Firestone Country Club in Akron, Ohio. Harrelson finished twenty-second and pocketed $210.

A Collision with Destiny

Raymond Earl "Ray" "Marion Mule" Fosse

Born: 1947
Cleveland Indians: 1967–72
Position: Catcher
Jersey Number: 8

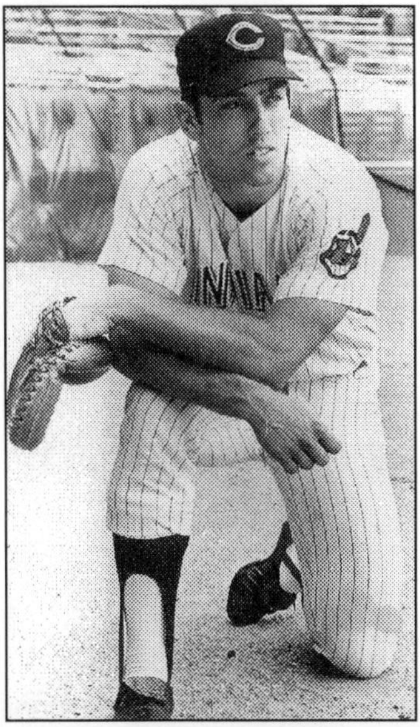

Ray Fosse, 1970 (Courtesy of the Williamson County Historical Society Museum)

SYMPTOMS

From 1960 until 1994, the best Tribe finish in the American League East was third place in 1968; even then, the team ended up 16.5 games out of first place. Attendance spiraled downward over the time, from a high of over 1.4 million in 1959, to nearly half that total for many of the subsequent years. Fans left much of their hope for postseason play at the plate and chose to follow individual stars and new prospects around the bases.

On June 8–9, 1965, Major League Baseball held its first amateur draft. Using the initial pick, the Kansas City Athletics chose an Arizona State player, Rick Monday. Cleveland, with the sixth pick, drafted an eighteen-year-old high school catcher who would become known as the "Marion Mule," Ray Fosse. Of the hitters drafted in the first round, Fosse went on to post the third-best number of at-bats at the major league level, behind only Monday and Bernie Carbo, who was taken by the Cincinnati Reds.

Fosse spent several years in the minors, ending up in 1968 at the Tribe's Triple-A affiliate, Portland. In 1969, he was called up late in the season and played in 37 games, batting a meager .172. The following year, everything changed for Fosse and the Cleveland baseball fans.

Fosse became the rock behind the plate during the early days of the 1970 season. On May 18, he was hitting .251, one of the three Tribe hitters who were batting over .250. Things seemed to gel when May ended. By June 22, Fosse was on a thirteen-game hitting streak. A few days later, on June 27, Fosse went 2–3, extending his streak to eighteen and raising his batting average to .313. In early July, Fosse's streak ended at twenty-three consecutive games. He was selected by Earl Weaver of the Baltimore Orioles as one of two Tribe representatives to take part in the All-Star Game at Riverfront Stadium in Cincinnati; Sam McDowell (see page 34) was the other player selected. Fosse had hit 16 home runs and batted in 45 runs by the All-Star break.

Fosse entered the July 14 All-Star Game in the fifth inning, replacing veteran Detroit Tiger catcher Bill Freehan. In the sixth inning, Fosse singled off of San Francisco right-hander Gaylord Perry and was driven in by Boston outfielder Carl Yastrzmeski. Fosse's next at bat came in the seventh inning, with men on second and third. The Cleveland catcher drove a ball to deep center field, scoring Baltimore's Brooks Robinson from third base.

With the score tied at 4–4, the contest went into extra innings. Both teams failed to get a run across the plate in the tenth or eleventh innings, and the American League hitters failed to produce a run in the twelfth. With two outs in the bottom of the twelfth, hometown hero Pete Rose—known as Charlie Hustle for his never-say-die style of play—singled and then moved to second on a single by Los Angeles Dodger infielder Billy Grabarkewitz. The scene was set for one of the most memorable collisions in baseball history, one that would undeservedly impact the Tribe's fortunes.

Chicago Cubs' Jim Hickman drove a pitch to center field. Speedy Kansas City Royal outfielder Amos Otis scooped up the ball while Rose rounded third, heading for home. Fosse positioned himself to block the plate, tracking Otis's throw. Rose chose not to slide, met Fosse before the ball arrived, and Fosse was sent sprawling as Rose scored the winning run. Whether Rose could have avoided Fosse is a question that is still debated today, but no one can doubt that Fosse's career went down like his body had from that point on. Later, Rose said he couldn't have faced his father if he hadn't hit Fosse hard.

Fosse played nine more years in the major leagues, winning two World Series rings with the Oakland A's in 1973 and 1974. Fosse played through his shoulder injury, diagnosed as a bad bruise, but actually a separation and fracture, and the lack of rest and treatment led to the decline in his power numbers. He never hit more than 12 home runs in a season and he ended his career with a total of 61 home runs.

Catchers are said to wear the "Tools of Ignorance," referring to the equipment—shin guards, chest protector and face mask—that hopefully shield the catcher from injury. The term means that the intelligence needed by a catcher to handle the duties of the position must be contrasted with the foolishness needed to play such a hazardous position. Fosse suffered a number of other injuries as well: a fracture of his right index finger, torn ligaments in his left hand, and a gash needing stitches on his right hand. His other serious injury occurred on June 5, 1974, when he broke up a clubhouse fight between Reggie Jackson and Billy North; Fosse suffered a disc injury in his neck, which landed him on the disabled list for three months. Fosse was traded back to Cleveland and played for them in 1976 and 1977. On May 30, 1977, Fosse caught Dennis Eckersley's no-hitter versus the California Angels and Eckersley gave him credit for calling a brilliant game. Fosse remained in baseball after retiring as a player and has served as the color analyst for the Oakland A's since 1986.

PATIENT HISTORY

"He is one of the finest young receivers I ever saw. You seldom see a ball get past him or even a dropped pitch. His arm is very strong and I think he can hit. He's big enough at 6–2 and 210 pounds."
—Walter Shannon, the Cleveland scout who signed Fosse

"He [Peter Rose] actually signed a baseball to me and wrote, 'To Ray. Thanks for making me famous.'"
—Ray Fosse

"And in Ray Fosse, who is only 23, we've got the best catcher in the league. I've been caught by Bill Freehan and John Roseboro and he's not far behind Cincinnati's John Bench in All-Star Games but I'm telling you Fosse is better."
—Sam McDowell, Cleveland pitcher

DIAGNOSIS

Ray Fosse was a preeminent catcher—smart, young, and tough. He was the player that the Indians of the 1970s could be built around. The Tribe fans hadn't seen a catcher like Fosse since Jim Hegan was behind the plate in the forties and fifties.

Fosse's injury at the 1970 All-Star Game took the wind out of the team's sails. While Fosse continued to play, he was clearly ailing. Rehabilitation and treatment for a separated shoulder were very different in 1970 than in the following decades. Fosse never regained his power stroke and, although he remained a good defensive catcher, there is no question that the shoulder injury cost Fosse a more decorated career. Cleveland fans thought Fosse had the potential to be another Johnny Bench, who helped lead Cincinnati to five National League pennants and two World Series championships.

Tribe followers despised Peter Rose for the collision with Fosse. Charlie Hustle had gone too far; Cleveland fans lost a rising star because

Rose took an unnecessary shot at Fosse in an exhibition game. Another before-the-injury dream became a depressing afterthought, contributing to the worst decade in Cleveland Indians baseball.

SECOND OPINION

After Fosse was traded, the Tribe lost more than leadership; home runs were down over the following seasons. The catching position was filled by the likes of Dave Duncan, Alan Ashby, Fred Kendall, and Gary Alexander. However, none of them could be mistaken for power hitters.

TREATMENT

Many medical and nonmedical professionals have trouble differentiating a separated shoulder from a dislocated shoulder. A separated shoulder (see medical illustration, page 298) is a widening or separation of the collarbone (clavicle) and the top of the shoulder blade (acromion), which can be seen on X-rays. The AC (acromion-clavicle) separation is also known as an AC sprain because the ligaments (the acromioclavicular (AC) and the coracoclavicular (CC) ligaments) between the two bones are injured or torn.

There are six types of separations. In a type I injury, the AC ligament is partially torn, but the CC ligament is not injured. In a type II injury, the AC ligament is completely torn, and the CC ligament is either not injured or partially torn and the collarbone is partially separated from the acromion. In a type III injury, both the AC and CC ligaments are completely torn and the collarbone and the acromion are completely separated.

There are three further classifications, types IV through VI, which are uncommon. These types of shoulder separations may involve tearing of the muscle that covers the upper arm and shoulder joint (deltoid muscle) and the one that extends from the back of the head, neck, and upper back across the back of the shoulder (trapezius muscle). Types I, II, and III generally heal well without surgery. The more significant tears need surgery.

The injury occurs after a fall or blow directly to the point or top of the shoulder. Fortunately, most sports-related separations are partial tears and respond well to early immobilization in a sling, followed by physical therapy. Athletes often return to play in four to six weeks, and injections are sometimes used to speed up recovery. The injury occurs most frequently in football, hockey, and wrestling, but is a risk in all sports. Long-term complications include chronic pain and early arthritis directly in the joint on the point of the shoulder.

INCIDENTAL FINDINGS

The Rose-Fosse collision might have been avoided if rule 7.13 was in place at the time. For the 2014 season, Major League Baseball and the Players' Association implemented the rule on an experimental basis. The rule reads:

> A runner attempting to score may not deviate from his direct pathway to the plate in order to initiate contact with the catcher (or other player covering home plate). If, in the judgment of the Umpire, a runner attempting to score initiates contact with the catcher (or other player covering home plate) in such a manner, the Umpire shall declare the runner out (even if the player covering home plate loses possession of the ball). In such circumstances, the Umpire shall call the ball dead, and all other base runners shall return to the last base touched at the time of the collision.
>
> Unless the catcher is in possession of the ball, the catcher cannot block the pathway of the runner as he is attempting to score. If, in the judgment of the Umpire, the catcher without possession of the ball blocks the pathway of the runner, the Umpire shall call or signal the runner safe. Notwithstanding the above, it shall not be considered a violation of this Rule 7.13

if the catcher blocks the pathway of the runner in order to field a throw, and the Umpire determines that the catcher could not have fielded the ball without blocking the pathway of the runner and that contact with the runner was unavoidable.

2.3 Million Reasons to Cry

Marcus Wayne Garland

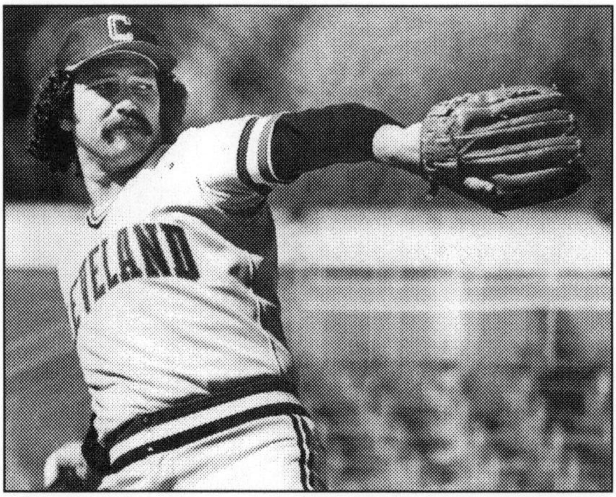

Born: 1950
Cleveland Indians: 1977–81
Position: Pitcher
Jersey Number: 17

Wayne Garland warming up during spring training, 1979 (*The Cleveland Press* Collection, Cleveland State University, Paul Tepley, photographer)

SYMPTOMS

Wayne Garland grew up as an All-American baseball prep star in Tennessee. He went on to attend Florida's Gulf Coast Junior College and had a 9–2 record with a 0.84 ERA in his last season there. In July 1969, the Baltimore Orioles signed him, giving him a bonus of over $30,000. He was brought up to the Orioles in 1973 and was mainly used out of the bullpen. Instead of re-signing with Baltimore in 1976 for the 1977 season, he chose to exercise his option to become a free agent after the season. Due to a thinned pitching roster, Garland was asked to start and compiled a 20–7 record, with an ERA of 2.67; he could now peddle his talents to the highest bidder.

After finishing fourth in 1976, the Cleveland Indians set their sights on Garland. Among the other free agents available were Sal Bando, Don Baylor, Rollie Fingers, Reggie Jackson, Joe Rudi, and Steve Stone. Clubs, not used to the new concept of free agency, were eager to spend money without completely understanding the ultimate value of their investments. Seeking a five-year, $1-million deal, Garland was shocked when the Indians offered him $2.3 million over ten years. He told his agent Jerry Kapstein that the deal was too good, but signing wouldn't be a problem.

Unfortunately, Garland injured his shoulder on a cold windy day in Tucson, Arizona, during his first spring training start with Cleveland. Diagnosed as bicipital tendonitis, several medical experts believed the injury was a result of Garland's 1976 season, when he pitched more than twice as many innings as he had previously. Garland tried to battle through the injury; he ultimately worked over 282 innings in 1977, losing 19 games along the way. He made just 6 starts in 1978 and 14 starts in 1979, with little success. The Indians released him after another injury-plagued season in 1981. Garland ended his Indians' career with 28 wins and 48 losses, and he never pitched professionally again.

PATIENT HISTORY

> "The guy is a killer.... He's the first guy I would compare with Catfish Hunter, and you don't just throw that kind of talk around."
> —Reggie Jackson

> "[I]n the length of time it took to write 'Wayne Garland' on the bottom line of a contract—Wayne Garland became a millionaire, and the Indians a pennant contender."
> —Russell Schneider, Cleveland sportswriter

> "When I stepped over the white line I gave 100 per cent every time. I'd much rather be known for that, because the contract is over with and I'm still here."
> —Wayne Garland

DIAGNOSIS

Wayne Garland was a big risk gone wrong, as the Cleveland Indians first attempted to battle the big market teams using free agency. In an effort to improve the atmosphere at Municipal Stadium and promote fan attendance, the Tribe brought in a promising young pitcher near the peak of his career. Unfortunately, Garland did not have a long record of success to justify the expense of his contract. Even if Garland had remained healthy, the team had overpaid.

Shoulder problems derailed Garland's once-promising career. While most said the injury was a result of overuse during his 20 win season, others said it happened due to an unseasonably cold day in Arizona. Regardless, the experience with Garland made the Indians reluctant to pursue free agents for a long time. The high contract costs also affected the Indians in their efforts to develop their own players.

To his credit, Garland worked hard to salvage something after the injury. He dutifully pitched game after game, with 38 starts despite the 19 losses in 1977. His play was limited to five partial seasons of his landmark ten-year contract.

As the Tribe continued to lose, the cavernous Municipal Stadium (capacity was a little over 78,000) felt like a mausoleum. Other than opening day, holidays, and when teams like the Yankees were in town, attendance was sparse. The Indians' players could feel the general apathy, which didn't help their morale or the ability to attract free agents.

SECOND OPINION

If Wayne Garland had posted a 19–13 record in 1977, the Tribe would have finished at 77–84 and fourth in the American League East. The Indians had no offense; the team finished ninth of fourteen teams in runs scored and seventh in batting average. The team also had little speed, finishing ninth in stolen bases.

The Tribe had been in the market for another free agent, Don Baylor, when they signed Garland. Baylor had also put up good numbers for the Orioles. He would end up a career .260 batter and average 24 home runs a season. His bat would have helped replace George Hendricks, who was traded to the San Diego Padres.

TREATMENT

The most common shoulder injury in overhead throwing athletes is known as impingement syndrome. The biggest, strongest muscles of the shoulder—which include the deltoid, the pectoralis, and the trapezius—are major support muscles for the shoulder. The "fine tuning" muscles, used when athletes attempt to serve in volleyball and tennis, throw a baseball, or swim are known as the rotator cuff muscles. In an overhead position, the rotator cuff muscle becomes pinched or impinged between the humerus bone and the acromion.

During the repetitive motion of throwing a baseball, the muscle and tendon of the rotator cuff can become inflamed, frayed, and ultimately torn (see medical illustration, page 299). The pitcher loses velocity, command of the strike zone, and strength. Although many athletes get better with rest and rehabilitation, the injury can require surgery in advanced cases. As the condition progresses, the tendon develops scar tissue and the resulting chronic pain can permanently affect an athlete's performance.

According to the Phillies' team physician Dr. Michael Ciccotti, rotator cuff surgery is not as successful as Tommy John surgery (see page 108). In part, Ciccotti attributes this to the fact that the UCL (Ulnar Collateral Ligament) in the elbow has a very good blood supply, which aids the healing process. Recent studies indicate that while pitchers can come back gradually over a three-year period from a torn rotator cuff, these pitchers typically did not perform as well as they did prior to their injury.

INCIDENTAL FINDINGS

While the name of Dr. Frank Jobe will be forever linked with Tommy John surgery, a less well-known figure who resided in Youngstown, Ohio, at the turn of the twentieth century was just as famous in the early years of baseball. John "Bonesetter" Reese and his orthopedic methods helped many injured ballplayers return to the diamond. Initially opposed by members of the medical profession, Reese finally was granted a license to practice his profession by the state of Ohio. As a youngster in his native Wales, Reese was trained by practical surgeons who were experts in the art of manipulation to correct deformities in the bony structure of the body. As his fame grew, his list of clients did as well; he treated Ty Cobb, Honus Wagner, Brooklyn shortstop Glenn Wright, and Cleveland outfielder Harry Bay.

Say It Ain't So Joe

Joseph "Super Joe" Charboneau

Born: 1955
Cleveland Indians: 1980–82
Position: Left Fielder/Designated Hitter
Jersey Number: 34

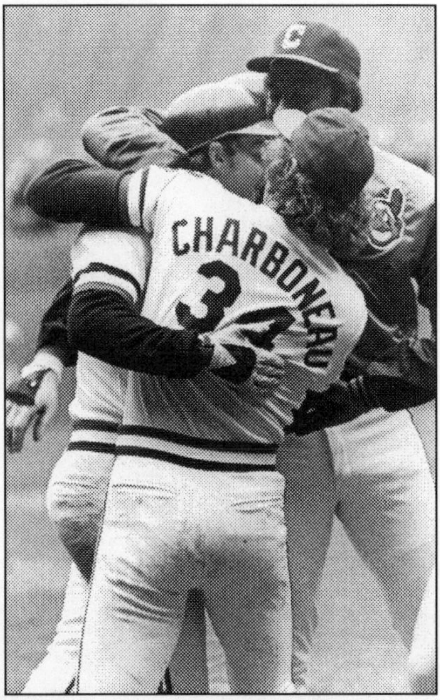

Joe Charboneau congratulates teammate, 1981. (*The Cleveland Press* Collection, Cleveland State University, photographer not known)

SYMPTOMS

In what the *Cleveland Plain Dealer* reported as a minor trade on December 7, 1978, the Indians acquired Phillies' farm hand Joe Charboneau for Cardell Camper, a pitching prospect. The twenty-one-year-old Charboneau had been playing in the California League, where he batted .350, with 18 home runs, 116 RBIs, and 119 runs scored. The Phillies had given up on the power hitter due to his propensity to get into bar fights and other eccentricities.

Charboneau spent the 1979 season with Chattanooga in the Double A Southern League before coming to Indians spring training in 1980. He got his break when Cleveland's first baseman Andre

Thornton required knee surgery in April. Mike Hargrove was moved to first base and Charboneau took over in left field. The rookie outfielder blasted a home run against the Angels on opening day, but "Super Joe" was truly christened during the Tribe's home opener, when he went three for three with three home runs. A few of his eccentricities that endeared him to the fans also were revealed—before games he took three vitamins in a specific order, got water from the same faucet, and rubbed his lucky charm, "Abernathy."

Charboneau ended the year with a .289 batting average, with 23 home runs and 87 RBIs. He was named the 1980 American League Rookie of the Year, the first Cleveland Indian to win the award since first baseman Chris Chambliss in 1971. Charboneau was the toast of the town; a song about the rookie charted at number four in the Cleveland market. A catchy little tune, the lyrics in part told the story of Super Joe.

> Who's the newest guy in town?
> Go Joe Charboneau.
> Turns the ballpark upside down.
> Go Joe Charboneau.
> Who do we appreciate?
> Go Joe Charboneau.
> (Song and Lyrics by Section 36)

Charboneau entered spring training in 1981, shouldering the hopes of a town and a team. During a preseason game, however, the outfielder injured his back. Examined on March 17, a first opinion recommended two weeks rest. A second opinion provided a different view—Joe was fine to resume spring training. After all, this was a guy who had broken his nose three times during his younger years while fighting in boxcars and warehouses for gamblers. He had tried to fix one of the breaks himself with a pair of pliers. This was the ballplayer who could drink beer through his nose (since the cartilage had been removed after another break), either by direct pour or by using a straw. This was "Super Joe."

The injury seemed to linger and Charboneau wasn't producing in the same way he had as a rookie. Hal Lebovitz, a prominent Cleveland sportswriter, was all too prescient in a story in the *Plain Dealer* on April 29, 1981. "I think Joe Charboneau's back is bothering him even though he tries to ignore the pain. The way he stooped for ground balls and threw in practice the other day indicated he was favoring his back and, if so, it has to be handicapping his swing."

In the strike-shortened 1981 season Charboneau was unproductive and ended up back in the minor leagues. After the season he underwent several back surgeries; all in all, parts of five discs were ultimately removed. "Super" Joe became "Subpar" Joe and never regained his 1980 form; he was out of the major leagues before the end of the 1982 season. After leaving the major leagues, Charboneau has been a college hitting coach, ran his own baseball academy, and has also worked for a local parks and recreation department.

PATIENT HISTORY

> "The guy is something else. No matter how we used him, he's come through."
> —Dave Garcia, Cleveland manager

> "He'd say, 'I don't know what's wrong. I just can't hit anymore. Will I ever be able to hit again?' Joe had lost all his confidence."
> —Cindi Charboneau

> "I love Cleveland. The city, the fans . . . you never know how long it will last."
> —Joe Charboneau

> "I don't mind saying that I'm bipolar. Baseball is a very structured event for me in my daily life. When I played, every day was structured."
> —Joe Charboneau

DIAGNOSIS

Joe Charboneau gave Cleveland fans a great thrill, unfortunately one that didn't last very long. He was Cleveland's Mark "The Bird" Fidrych or the fictional Joe Hardy from "Damn Yankees." Charboneau was the quintessential one-hit (or in his case one-season) wonder. His career ended so quickly that fans felt the 1980 season had been a dream. For one fleeting year, Charboneau had brought back memories of Rocky Colavito.

Of all of Super Joe's accomplishments, Cleveland fans remember one in particular. In a June game against the Yankees during his magical season, Charboneau blasted a majestic homer into the third deck on a pitch from Yankee starter Tom Underwood. At the time, no player had hit a home run into the third deck of the remodeled Yankee stadium; Jimmie Fox and Frank Howard had sent homers into the third deck of the old Yankee stadium.

During Super Joe's great season, the Tribe finished sixth. Joe was a distraction and a good one; he brought entertainment to a fan base that hoped the Indians wouldn't be mathematically eliminated from postseason play by the All-Star break. Cleveland needed a weird character to lessen the disappointment of a baseball team headed for the cellar. If nothing else, for one glorious year Charboneau filled that purpose. He never filled it again, because his baseball career "fell off of a cliff," but his antics and heroics made him a quasi-celebrity, one fondly remembered by Cleveland fans.

SECOND OPINION

Charboneau's impact was short-lived and his power numbers would have helped the Tribe in the following years. During Charboneau's breakout season, the Tribe's ERA was 4.68. Two years later, the Indians' hurlers allowed one-half runs less per contest. Without Charboneau, the Tribe scored 50 less runs in 1982.

TREATMENT

In 1991, Neurosurgical Clinics in North America developed a new name to describe certain types of back pain. Failed Back Surgery Syndrome (FBSS) or Failed Back Syndrome (FBS) refers to long-term back or leg pain that occurs after spinal surgery.

Many factors contribute to the development of FBSS or FBS, including recurrent disc herniation (slippage), spinal canal narrowing (stenosis), persistent nerve pressure, scar tissue, anxiety, sleeplessness, depression, and muscle weakness. Treatment includes physical therapy, pain medication, TENS (transcutaneous electrical nerve stimulation), nerve blocks, and implantable medicine pumps. For this reason, spine surgeons usually explore other treatment options before surgery. In the last twenty years, treatment alternatives for chronic back pain have dramatically improved. Pain clinics are common places for patients to seek care before or after FBSS or FBS.

INCIDENTAL FINDINGS

By all accounts, Super Joe was not your average guy. After his career he indicated he had bipolar disorder. Perhaps his injury upset his routine and hindered his recovery.

In studies of FBS patients, it has been noted that psychological, social, and behavioral "issues play a significant role in the outcome of the surgery as well, since patients with chronic low back pain as a result of FBS frequently have psychological illnesses. These psychopathologies include depressive disorders, anxiety, and somatization, all of which may be undertreated. A patient's psychopathology is thought to influence the pain level and outcome from aggressive spine surgeries" (Daniel Aghion, Pradeep Chopra, and Adetokunbo A. Oyelese, "Failed Back Syndrome," *Rhode Island Medical Journal* no. 12, December 2012).

Straining the Fans' Backs

Keith Hernandez

Born: 1953
Cleveland Indians: 1990
Position: First Baseman
Jersey Number: 17

SYMPTOMS

In December 1989, the Indians signed thirty-seven-year-old Keith Hernandez to a contract that awarded the aging first baseman a guaranteed $3.5 million for two years. Due to injury, Hernandez had played less than 100 games in 1988 and 1989. The Tribe finished in sixth place in 1989 and Hernandez was brought in to solidify the infield and provide leadership for a team that had fallen apart in the latter months of the previous season. To make room for the Mets first baseman, the team's power hitter Joe Carter was traded to the San Diego Padres for three players. Two of the players from that trade, Sandy Alomar and Carlos Baerga, would become part of the pennant-winning and World Series contending teams of the mid-1990s and early 2000s. Hernandez would be long gone by then.

Hernandez was a five-time All-Star and won the National League MVP award in 1979. That year, as a St. Louis Cardinal, he led the league with a .349 batting average and scored 116 runs. In 1982, Hernandez was part of St. Louis' World Series victory. After being traded to the New York Mets, Hernandez was a vital cog in the team's 1986 World Series crown.

During spring training in 1990, Hernandez complained of a back issue. It was an old injury, one that he had had prior to coming to the Indians; he had been seeing a chiropractor once a week for treatment. Hernandez began the season, but near the end of May he suffered a calf injury, described as either a strain or tear. He was placed on the disabled list twice more that season; he played only 43 games, batted .200, and hit one home run. The following year he didn't play in any games and then retired. In the end, Hernandez received almost $27,000 for each of his plate appearances. Paying Hernandez didn't leave much cash for bargaining in the free agent market, and in 1991, the last year of Hernandez's contract, the Tribe finished in seventh place with a record of 57–105.

PATIENT HISTORY

> "It's still baseball, and I feel we [Cleveland Indians] have a better ball club than people give us credit for. I think we're going to be a surprise."
> —Keith Hernandez

> "Having Keith is like having an insurance policy. He knows the pitchers. He knows the hitters. He knows all the subtleties, and he does not keep them to himself."
> —Wally Backman, New York Mets

> "[H]e traded himself. He wasn't hustling... he would sit in the clubhouse doing crossword puzzles. He must have been awfully good at puzzles."
> —White Herzog, St. Louis Cardinals' Manager

DIAGNOSIS

The Cleveland Indians signed Keith Hernandez before the start of the 1990 season, hoping he would add a veteran presence to a young team. The Indians had experienced a miserable 1989 season and wanted to shore up first base defensively; they believed that Hernandez could fill that role. His signing, however, was a case of picking up a player not a year too late, but rather several years too late. Hernandez represented the downward spiral of Cleveland teams in the

1980s and early 1990s, one that would paradoxically result in the greatest baseball renaissance in Indians' history.

Cleveland fans were originally enraged with what turned out to be a significant waste of $3.5 million. Later in the season, fans were still upset, but by the time Hernandez had surgery and mostly disappeared, fan apathy had set in. Fans questioned his motives, knowing he would rather be in New York. The spine surgery, reportedly to fix a disc injury, confirmed the inevitable for Indians fans. Bad luck with an injury, a waste of money with a bad contract, and a hole at first base contributed to the worst record in team history. For fans of the Cleveland Indians, that's saying a lot.

SECOND OPINION

If the Indians were looking to improve defensively at first base, Hernandez had several Gold Gloves to prove his value as a fielder. Still, comparing their careers, Pete O'Brien, the Tribe's first baseman in 1989, fielded just as well as Hernandez. O'Brien, five years younger than Hernandez, was a free agent after the 1989 season. Perhaps the Tribe didn't want to invest in him, though the Indians' front office paid about $500,000 more for Hernandez. O'Brien ended up signing with the Mariners.

Even with Hernandez playing in only 42 games, the Tribe's batting average rose from thirteenth (out of fourteen teams) in 1989 to second. However, pitching took a dive. In 1989, the Tribe had a respectable 3.65 ERA and was fifth in the league. The following year, the Indians' hurlers posted a dismal 4.26 ERA (thirteenth in the league). Like many other seasons, the Tribe was active in the pennant race, if trading players to contenders was the measuring stick.

TREATMENT

Back pain and disc injuries (see medical illustration, page 301) are common in athletes, but also in the general adult population. The disc is a round, shock-absorbing pad found between each of the bony vertebrae. A slipped disc is a misleading term for an injury where the round (annular) ligament containing the soft disc tears, allowing the disk to bulge, slip, or wear out prematurely. A disc is surrounded by many nerve endings, so a slipped disc can cause great pain. A disc also can put pressure on nerves that exit the back; nerve irritation, inflammation, or entrapment can lead to pain or numbness in the hamstrings, the calf, or even the foot and ankle. A disc is prone to tearing or rupturing from persistent loading or twisting of the trunk, making the injury common in sports that emphasize trunk rotation (e.g., swinging a baseball bat).

Lumbar discs, which affect the lower back, often improve greatly with noninvasive treatment. Noninvasive treatment options include medicine, physical therapy, manipulation, injections, and rest. Athletes are frequently left with some deficit, especially when the disc develops a degenerative disk space, that is, becomes a worn-out shock absorber. The loss of disk space might appear as bone (vertebrae) on bone on a routine x-ray. To evaluate the extent of injury more accurately, a MRI is useful. In some athletes, surgery may be necessary to take pressure off a nerve in the back. In the last ten years, noninvasive techniques have improved and a smaller percentage of athletic disc injuries need surgery.

INCIDENTAL FINDINGS

In the late 1800s and early 1900s, baseball players travelled the country primarily via the rails. Train accidents were not uncommon and a malady arose called "railway spine." Injured passengers sued for damages. Medical experts, hired by insurers, found no outward injuries and testified that railway spine was a hysterical state. Patients who claimed that they had severe pain in their legs and backs were deemed fakers. Undoubtedly, many injuries were caused by the sudden and violent rotation of the back when rail cars derailed or crashed into others trains, but medical technology wasn't mature enough to detect internal injuries.

Shouldering the Blame

Kenneth "Kenny" Lofton

Born: 1967
Cleveland Indians: 1992–2007
Position: Center Fielder
Jersey Number: 7

SYMPTOMS

Kenny Lofton, raised by his grandmother in a tough Chicago-area neighborhood, was a high school basketball star for East Chicago (Indiana) Washington and accepted a scholarship to the University of Arizona. Lofton was the sixth man on a Wildcat squad that reached the Final Four in 1988 and started at point guard for the 1989 team, which was frequently ranked first in the polls.

Lofton did play baseball briefly at Arizona and was drafted by the Houston Astros in 1988. By 1991, Lofton had made it to Triple A, where he batted .308, with 93 runs and 40 steals. In December of that year, the Indians sent a promising catcher Ed Taubensee and pitcher Willie Blair to Houston for Lofton. The deal turned out to be one of the best ones the Tribe ever made.

In eight years with the Indians (Lofton did make a brief return to the Tribe in 2007), Lofton had a .311 average, stole 431 bases, and was a defensive mainstay in center field. He was selected for the All-Star team six times and won four Gold Gloves. Lofton sparked a team that won the American League Central Division title six times (they also finished first in 2007).

Lofton and his teammates were favored to win the 1999 World Series. They finished the regular season in first place with a record of 97–65, and faced the Red Sox (94–68), who had finished second to the New York Yankees in the American League East. After winning the first two games in the best of five series, the Indians lost the next two in Boston.

The deciding game five was played at Jacobs Field (now Progressive Field) in front of a sold-out throng. By the middle of the fourth inning, the score was tied at 8–8 in a slugfest. In the bottom of the fourth, the Indians suffered what the *Akron Beacon Journal* called "Another Strange Twist of Fortune" (October 12, 1999). With one out, Lofton hit a sharp grounder to first. Hoping to beat the throw to pitcher Pedro Martinez, who was covering the base, Lofton slid headfirst into the bag. He was called out and he was out of the game with a dislocated shoulder. As Indians second baseman Roberto Alomar said, "It seemed like everything after that [Lofton's injury] went numb. Everybody went quiet. Nobody knew what happened. But after that, it seemed like we couldn't do nothing" (*Akron Beacon Journal*, October 12, 1999). Boston scored four more runs and Cleveland lost the playoff and any hope of winning a World Series.

PATIENT HISTORY

> "He's got a chance to be the type of center fielder you look for in a major leaguer."
> —Reggie Waller, Auburn Astros Manager

> "There are certain players you know have talent and they give it to you every time out. . . . I never walked away from the ballpark without being excited for what Kenny Lofton gave me."
> —John Hart, Cleveland General Manager

> "We were part of something special, moving into the new ballpark (in 1994) and the fans responding. We knew it had been a thousand years since they made the playoffs and we were proud to be part of it [playoff and World Series runs]."
> —Kenny Lofton

DIAGNOSIS

Watching Cleveland Indians baseball was fun in the 1990s; the team was great and the crowds were raucous. Kenny Lofton was one of several Indians players worth the price of admission. The quality baseball during the 1990s led to one of the great records in Cleveland sports history—455 straight sellouts in snow, during near rain-outs, and at midweek snoozers. Sadly, the team could not bring home the elusive World Series crown. Lofton's injury (even little leaguers are taught not to slide head first into first base) in the deciding game of 1999 spoiled the team's last chance to win a World Series during that halcyon era.

SECOND OPINION

Lofton's injury undoubtedly had an effect on the fifth game outcome, but more important were the failure of the Tribe's bullpen and the lack of hitting against Boston hurler Pedro Martinez. Martinez followed Bret Saberhagen and Derek Lowe, who were ineffective, and pitched six shutout innings. Tribe reliever Paul Shuey gave up three runs in the seventh, which sealed the Tribe's fate.

In the following two seasons, Lofton's batting average dropped and he eventually signed as a free agent with the Chicago White Sox. Still, the Tribe was a respectable 90–72 in 2000, finishing second in the American League Central; the team scored the second most runs in the league. The following season, the Indians finished first with a record of 91–71, losing to the Seattle Mariners in the first round of American League Division Series. From 1999 to 2001, the Tribe's pitching staff saw their ERA rise from sixth in the league to ninth. The Seattle series was a microcosm of the Tribe's saga—they could outhit teams and win, but in close games, their pitching wasn't up to the task.

TREATMENT

The shoulder joint, like the knee joint, is two distinct and vastly different joints. The acromioclavicular joint is at the top, or point, of the shoulder and this joint is the stable protector of the ball and socket joint below it. The glenohumeral joint, the ball and socket that looks like a large golf ball on a tee in X-rays, provides great freedom of movement in all directions, more so than other joints like the knee, ankle, and hip. During the extremes of sporting activity, the ball can slip partly away from the tee (sublux) or slip completely off the tee (dislocate), resulting in a broken bone, torn ligament (capsule), or torn cartilage (glenoid labrum tear).

A separated shoulder (acromioclavicular [AC] separation or sprain) is an injury to the ligaments that hold the collarbone to the shoulder blade (see medical illustration, page 298). In a mild separated shoulder, the ligaments may just be stretched. In severe injuries, ligaments may be completely torn. A separated shoulder is usually treated by means of a sling or shoulder immobilizer, which keeps the patient from lifting her/his arm away from the chest and helps the ligaments heal.

A dislocated shoulder is an injury where the upper arm bone pops out of the cup-shaped socket that is part of the shoulder blade (see medical illustration, page 300). A dislocated shoulder is a more extensive injury than a separated shoulder. A dislocated shoulder requires treatment by a trained medical professional to reduce (put back into place) the shoulder. Surgery is sometimes necessary following a dislocated shoulder if there has been extensive damage to muscles, tendons, nerves, blood vessels, or the labrum, or if dislocations are recurrent. Athletes who suffer these shoulder injuries can experience looseness and weakness, adversely affecting performance.

INCIDENTAL FINDINGS

The Indians did acquire another player in the Kenny Lofton trade. The other player, David Grant Rohde, isn't a household name in

Cleveland. Coincidently, the two players were at the University of Arizona in 1986. Rohde helped the Wildcats win the 1986 College World Series. When Rohde showed up in Cleveland, he probably was quite familiar with the Tribe's spring training facilities. After all, he had played at Hi Corbett Field when he was at Arizona. The Tribe used the facilities from 1946–92. Rohde practiced there as an Indian for only one year.

A Tragic End for Cleveland Fans

Steven Robert Olin

Born: 1965 Died: 1993
Cleveland Indians: 1990–92
Position: Pitcher
Jersey Number: 31

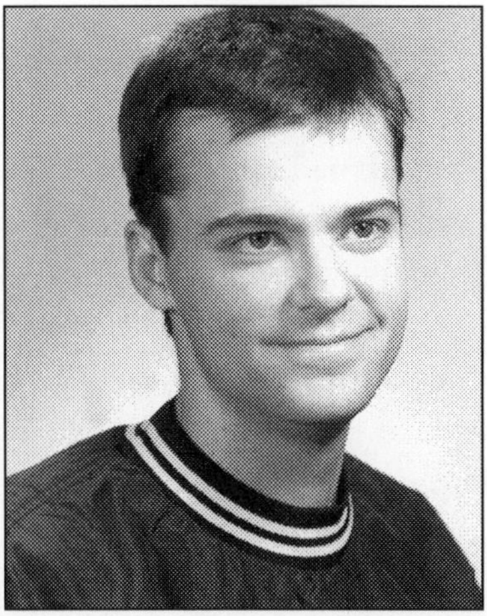

Steve Olin, Portland State University, 1986 (Courtesy Athletic Department, Portland State University)

Stanley Timothy "Tim" Crews

Born: 1961 Died: 1993
Cleveland Indians: Never played in a regular season game
Position: Pitcher
Jersey Number: N/A

Robert Michael "Bob" Ojeda

Born: 1957
Cleveland Indians: 1993
Position: Pitcher
Jersey Number: 17

SYMPTOMS

Steve Olin's best, and unfortunately last year in baseball, 1989, coincided with the Indians' hiring of Mike Hargrove as manager. Olin, a submarining right-handed reliever, became the Tribe's closer, posting 27 saves. The twenty-six-year-old pitcher had come up in 1989, a season the Indians finished second to last. By 1992, Cleveland had moved up to fourth place and had a core of young players ready to compete for a pennant.

Tim Crews, a Dodgers free agent, was signed by the Tribe in January 1993. Crews was primarily a middle-reliever and had been part of the Dodgers' World Series winning team. His arrival was intended to bolster the bullpen, provide spot starts when needed, and allow him to become a vocal leader in the clubhouse. Crews suffered a broken rib during a spring training drill, but that wasn't the reason he never played a regular season game for Cleveland.

Bob Ojeda was in his late thirties when he was signed as a free agent by the Tribe in December 1992. Ojeda had played for Boston, the Mets, and the Dodgers over a thirteen-year career. He had been a key cog in the 1986 New York Mets World Series victory. The left-hander was to fill one of the Indians' starting pitcher positions. In the end, he only started seven games and pitched forty-eight innings in 1993, pitched three innings the following year for the Yankees, and retired from the game.

On March 22, 1993, Ojeda and Olin joined Tim and Laurie Crews at their new ranch twenty-five miles outside Orlando, Florida, on the only off day from spring training that year. A fishing party originally planned for the afternoon was delayed by rain. The three ballplayers went out after dark on Little Lake Nellie on Crews' eighteen-foot bass boat. Returning to shore, the boat sped into a wooden pier at about 60 mph, killing Olin, twenty-seven, instantly. The next morning, Crews, thirty-one, died from his injuries at a hospital in Orlando. Ojeda, thirty-five, suffered lacerations on the head and lost two quarts of blood, but survived.

Ojeda later said he didn't remember hitting the pier; everything just seemed gray, but he could feel and smell blood. Ojeda would return in August after physical rehabilitation and mental therapy to combat survivor's guilt. Needless to say, the Indians organization was saddened and stunned. Instead of concentrating on baseball, the team had to bury two players and answer media questions about the accident. The team finished the season in second to last place at 76–86.

PATIENT HISTORY

> "It changed the whole team, the whole chemistry. We never recovered because of the way it happened."
> —Sandy Alomar

> "The thing I remember most about Tim [Crews] was his daily joy in wearing a major-league uniform. I don't know anybody who was more liked by his teammates. I don't know anybody who got more out of their ability."
> —Fred Claire, former Dodgers general manager

> "I tried to clear my eyes and realized that part of my forehead had fallen over them like a trap door."
> —Bobby Ojeda

DIAGNOSIS

By 1993, it was clear that the Cleveland Indians were building momentum. The Indians had improved by 19 wins in 1992, finishing in fourth place, with a record of 76–86. A nucleus of young players was growing together as the Indians prepared to play their last season in the cavernous Municipal Stadium. The excitement surrounding the new stadium was tangible as the beautiful new crown jewel took shape in downtown Cleveland.

In the meantime, local favorite Mike Hargrove was molding an impressive daily lineup that included Sandy Alomar, Albert Belle, Carlos Baerga, Kenny Lofton, and Jim Thome. The pitching staff was a work in progress, but Steve Olin, a young relief pitcher, was gaining confidence right along with the everyday lineup. Olin looked like he would play a major role in the team's revival, whether as a late inning matchup righty, or as the team's closer. The Indians added a veteran presence in 1993 by bringing in Tim Crews and Bob Ojeda as free agents.

The spring training tragedy knocked the wind out of Cleveland sports fans. Mike Hargrove struggled to keep the young team together, as painful memories of Little Lake Nellie dimmed the team's play for the entire season. In some ways, the tragedy tarnished the transition of Cleveland Indians baseball from Municipal Stadium to Jacobs Field.

Later in the 1990s, Tribe fans experienced joy and passion not seen in Cleveland for decades. The team was dominant, Jacobs Field was the crown jewel of baseball, and fans filled the stadium in record numbers. One question remained; could the Indians have won a championship with Steve Olin as the closer? José Mesa was brilliant at times, but his inconsistency was a problem, especially during the 1997 World Series.

SECOND OPINION

The unfortunate accident eventually led to José Mesa becoming the Tribe's closer. Mesa, a two-time All-Star and Cy Young runner-up, was by all accounts a very productive closer. Olin, in his one season as the Tribe's late-inning reliever, gave up on average one hit per inning pitched and averaged less than one strikeout per inning pitched. It's true that Mesa's postseason record was hardly stellar, but part of the reason the Tribe was playing in October was Mesa's April through September numbers.

TREATMENT

According to a Center for Disease Control report (2010), an estimated 1.7 million people sustain a traumatic brain injury (TBI) annually. Most are the result of a fall of some type. Newer treatments have reduced the number of deaths from TBI. Over the past thirty years, deaths from severe TBI have been reduced from 50 percent to fewer than 25 percent.

The symptoms of TBI can be classified into three broad categories. Physical symptoms can include seizures, paralysis, dizziness, tremors, and balance issues. Cognitive symptoms can effect concentration, processing speed, memory, and learning. Behavioral symptoms, such as anxiety, sleep problems, mood swings, and temper outbursts are not uncommon.

New treatment protocols take into account these challenges. Since TBI does not manifest itself similarly in all patients, treatment must take this factor into account. After stabilizing the patient, medications might be administered to minimize secondary damage to the brain or surgery might be required. In most cases, periods of rehabilitation will also be required to help patients relearn basic skills and return to daily activities.

INCIDENTAL FINDINGS

Survivor's guilt is a deep feeling of guilt often experienced by those who have survived some catastrophe that took the lives of others. Ojeda felt the impact of his teammates' deaths and he showed classic symptoms of survivor's guilt—after the accident he went to Stockholm, Sweden, without telling anyone, he withdrew from his family, he experienced nightmares, he changed his diet, couldn't sleep, and had recurring memories of the accident brought on by little things, like the smell of coffee or riding a ferry in Seattle.

Luckily, he received therapy and was able to return to baseball, although briefly. His recovery was not simple or quick, as with most cases of survivor's guilt. Continued reassurance from his doctor and the families of the deceased players provided help at critical times.

Bad News Travels Fast

Jaret Samuel Wright

Born: 1975
Cleveland Indians: 1997–2002
Position: Pitcher
Jersey Number: 27

SYMPTOMS

Jaret Wright—the son of Clyde Wright, who pitched for the California Angels during his major-league career—was a baseball and football star in high school. He possessed an over-powering fastball and with his arm strength made a very good quarterback. Unlike many high school signal callers, Wright had the size of a fullback, standing six foot one and weighing 215 pounds.

The Cleveland Indians drafted Wright out of high school with the tenth overall pick in 1994. Wright's fastball had reportedly been clocked at 98 mph and he was paid a signing bonus of $1.2 million, the most the Tribe had ever paid a rookie. He reported to the Burlington Indians of the Appalachian League and quickly worked his way up to Triple A. After an injury to Tribe starter Jack McDowell in June 1997, Wright was called up and made his pitching debut on June 24. Despite giving up five runs and seven hits in 5 2/3 innings, he was credited with the 10–5 win over the Twins. The Tribe went on to finish second behind the White Sox, but won the American League Division Series against the Yankees and won the American League Championship Series over the Orioles. Unfortunately, the Indians lost the World Series in seven games to the Florida Marlins.

Wright was pivotal in the Indians' 1997 postseason run. He won two games, including the deciding fifth game against the Yankees. He pitched game four against the Orioles, a series the Tribe eventually won. In the World Series he won game four and pitched six scoreless innings in game seven, only to see the bullpen fail to hold the lead.

The Indians made the playoffs in 1998, but Wright had a mediocre year, going 12–10 with a disappointing 4.72 ERA. Some experts said Wright was relying too heavily on his fastball. Once hitters knew it was coming, they could adjust and hit it. Wright performed poorly in the 1998 postseason, but the Indians' brass still considered Wright to be a major part of the team's future.

Wright came out of spring training in good shape in 1999 and the Tribe was looking to make another run at the World Series. In July, Wright was pulled from a game against the Houston Astros after five innings, complaining of soreness in his shoulder. During the outing, his dominant fastball was clocked at less than 90 mph. The team's orthopedist called the injury a problem in the rhomboid region (muscles in the upper back). He was placed on the fifteen-day disabled list. The following year, Wright needed surgery and rehabilitation. Wright was never able to dominate with his fastball, the Tribe didn't re-sign him, and he became a free agent. His best post-Indians year was in 2004 with Atlanta, when he won fifteen games; his major league career ended in 2007.

Jaret had all "The Wright Stuff." He had the arm strength and attitude to be a long-term Indians starter. But his shoulder injury and subsequent surgeries made his fall to earth all too quick.

PATIENT HISTORY

> "[H]e was exposed to the Big League atmosphere growing up. I see the same arrogance and belief in himself that I saw in his dad [Clyde Wright], but I see a lot better stuff."
> —Mike Hargrove, Cleveland Manager

> "You just don't see kids with an arm like that. But he [Wright] does need a curve ball."
> —Bob Feller

> "He's as good as I've seen in twelve years of scouting. I haven't seen a high school player throw as hard as Jaret...he throws 90–92 (miles per hour), and I've seen him get up to 95–98 with men on base."
>
> —Jay Robertson, Indians Scouting Director

DIAGNOSIS

Wright came to Cleveland during the rebirth of baseball on the shores of Lake Erie. Cleveland Indians fans, burdened with forty years of disappointment, seemed to be on the threshold of a dream season. Wright appeared to be the ace the Tribe needed in the starting rotation, which included twenty-four-year-old Bartolo Colon and thirty-year-old Charles Nagy, to push the team over the top.

The twenty-one-year-old rookie phenom, featuring a strong major league baseball pedigree, had opened the season as the starter for the Tribe's AA Akron affiliate, but finished the year on the mound in Florida against the Marlins in the seventh game of the World Series. The dream of winning it all was shattered in the most painful of endings when the Tribe gave up a 2–1 lead in the ninth inning before losing in the eleventh. Wright, though, had pitched one-run baseball into the seventh inning.

The Indians had great hopes for many more World Series after uncovering a gem in Wright. His value was through the roof after his rookie season, and rumors surfaced that Pedro Martinez, the Cy Young award winner, was available in a trade for Wright. However, the Indians never made it back to the fall classic, and Wright's talent disappeared after multiple shoulder injuries, chronic pain issues, and surgeries. Did he pitch too much and too soon? Was there a flaw in his delivery? Cleveland fans were left to wonder "what if," and Wright left Cleveland without a World Series ring.

SECOND OPINION

The year after Wright came on the postseason scene, the Tribe's ERA was even better than in 1997; Wright was only 12–10. Unfortunately, the Tribe batters weren't as productive. Even though the team finished first, the Indians' finished sixth in batting average and runs. The previous year they were third in both categories.

The following two seasons, the Tribe finished second and first in batting average and first and second in runs scored, respectively, but pitching suffered. In 1999, the Cleveland staff had an ERA of 4.89 (sixth out of fourteen teams) and in 2000 the ERA was 4.84 (seventh out of fourteen teams). Jaret Wright's pitching prowess was as short-lived as Joe Charboneau's home run swing.

TREATMENT

In 2000, the Tribe reported that Wright had a torn labrum and minor fraying of the rotator cuff (see medical illustration, page 299). He had surgery that year and again in 2001. Later in his career, he missed time with a shoulder strain and inflammation of the shoulder.

Four common problems can cause a shoulder injury.

1. Impingement (pinching) of the rotator cuff or bursal sac under the bony and ligament attachment of the collar bone (clavicle) and shoulder blade (acromion). The injury occurs when an athlete raises his arm overhead such as in the motion of pitching a baseball and is classified as an overuse injury.
2. Recurrent dislocation occurs when the ball (humerus) of the upper arm slips out of the socket (glenoid rim) due to a tear of the supportive shock absorber (glenoid labrum) or supportive ligaments (capsule).
3. Painful instability (looseness) occurs when the arm is forced beyond its normal range of motion. The ball moves abnormally on the socket.

4. Osteoarthritis (wear and tear) destroys the smooth outer covering (articular cartilage) of bone. This wearing down is caused by abnormal motion of the ball and socket or trauma to the acromioclavicular (collar bone/shoulder blade) joint on point of the shoulder. Athletes can have worn cartilage or loose bodies of bone or cartilage with arthritis.

Four common surgical procedures can be performed to alleviate shoulder injuries.

1. Arthroscopy surgery allows the surgeon to look into the joint with a small, pencil-sized telescope and to work through another small incision in the skin. This technique causes minimal damage to muscles and skin, allowing for shorter recovery times. Techniques have evolved since the mid-1990s and continue to improve.
2. Bankart repair surgery tightens ligaments and repairs the capsule and the glenoid labrum in an attempt to improve shoulder movement and prevent recurrent dislocations and instability or looseness.
3. Rotator cuff repair surgery repairs a torn tendon to improve the function of the shoulder joints and the muscles that move the shoulder. This procedure can be done open (requiring a several centimeter long incision) or arthroscopically.
4. Shoulder replacement surgery is indicated for badly worn out shoulders. The ball is replaced or resurfaced to improve movement. The surgery has become more widely available in the last ten years.

Surgery is followed by physical therapy to restore normal range of motion and strength to damaged muscles and tendons. A shoulder surgery fails if it does not achieve the expectations of the surgeon or the athlete. Failure can result from stiffness, weakness, instability, pain, or failure to heal from complications, such as infection or nerve injuries. The expectations for athletes are higher, especially for professional pitchers. Throwing a baseball is a complex movement and to return to competitive pitching at the major league level is very difficult. This makes surgery extremely challenging, even in the most ideal circumstances.

INCIDENTAL FINDINGS

Using up a pitcher's arm is a very real concern for most managers. Teams sometimes "shut down" a young starter after he has pitched a certain number of innings in a given season. These actions might go out the window when a World Series is at stake, but saving a promising prospect is as old as the game.

> The young twirler is cautioned not to use curves for the first few days, but simply pitches straight balls. Pitching a curve is a great strain on the muscles of the arms and if performed without proper preparation, may ruin the career of a promising twirler. The arm is not in condition to be twisted in any way, and a sudden snap of that member, such as is employed in throwing a curve, may displace the sinews, and cause great pain. This will disappear after a while, but the player may never again be able to pitch as well as before. His arm will be practically dead, and he will have what is known as a glass arm. The pitcher may be a great player, but five or six innings will be his limit. Unless the real injury is discovered he will have to retire from baseball. (*Physical Culture* 23, 1910)

The Second Time Isn't a Charm

Juan Alberto "Juan Gone" González

Born: 1969
Cleveland Indians: 2001 and 2005
Position: Outfielder
Jersey Number: 22 (2001) and 16 (2005)

SYMPTOMS

In 2004, the Tribe finished in third place with a record 80–82. Although their record was below .500, the Indians had a good core of pitchers led by Cliff Lee, C. C. (Carsten Charles) Sabathia, and Jake Westbrook. After signing Atlanta pitcher Kevin Milwood in the off-season, the Tribe decided to bring back the thirty-five-year-old Juan González to bolster the offense. González had played for the Tribe in 2001, signing a one-year, $11-million contract, and batted .325, with 35 home runs and 140 RBIs.

González's career started in 1989 with the Texas Rangers and he became, by most accounts, the best run producer the team ever had. The slugger also played briefly for Detroit and Kansas City. Prior to signing with Cleveland after the 2004 season, González was plagued by back and hamstring injuries, playing in 70 games in 2002, 82 games in 2003, and 33 games in 2004.

González's career statistics are Hall of Fame caliber. Unfortunately, the outfielder played in baseball's "steroid era." Although the evidence of González's steroid use is mostly circumstantial, he was heavily implicated in Jose Canseco's book, the exposé that detailed baseball's rampant substance abuse. Also, after he left Texas a piece of González's luggage was snared at the Cleveland airport because it contained performance-enhancing drugs and steroid paraphernalia. Mention of González's name was also very prominent in the Mitchell report that investigated illicit drug use in baseball (see page 97).

While the Indians' signing of González was considered a low risk—$600,000 for making the opening day roster with additional incentive clauses—the Tribe was hopeful the aging slugger had one more good year left in his bat. During spring training, González suffered a left hamstring strain and after returning he strained his right hamstring. He remained in an extended spring training program in Winter Haven, Florida, until mid-May, when he went to Triple-A Buffalo. Called up in late May, he was inserted into the starting lineup against the Twins at the Metrodome. In his first at bat, he grounded to third base and strained his right hamstring running to first. "Juan Gone" left the game and major league baseball. His career was over.

PATIENT HISTORY

"Juan's always got a smile. He just loves to play baseball."
—Charlie Manuel, Tribe manager

"I have nothing to hide. Nothing. And I offered to be tested, whenever they wanted. If you have nothing to hide, there is nothing to worry about."
—Juan González

"He's the kind of guy who you'll look back on and say 'It was an honor playing with him.'"
—Dean Palmer, Texas third baseman

DIAGNOSIS

The Indians were desperate for a right-handed power hitter in 2005. There was hope that González would catch lightening in a bottle again, like he had in 2001. Unfortunately, in his much-anticipated debut he suffered a significant hamstring tear in his first and only at bat with the team that season. Later that season, the Indians became one of the hottest teams in baseball and made a run at the playoffs after winning 44 out of 60 games, including an 18–2 stretch in September. The young Indians lost three straight games to the Kansas City Royals and Tampa Bay Devil Rays, however, and lost control of the division title. The Tribe missed out on the Wild Card on the last day of the season, despite ending the year with a 93–69 record. Even a partially healthy Juan González could have taken the Indians into the post-season as a team whose pitching staff would have been dominant.

SECOND OPINION

Juan González might have made a difference if he had stayed healthy. Without him, the Tribe still performed extremely well. The team led the American League with a 3.61 ERA; the problem seemed to be clutch hitting. In 2004, the Tribe hit 184 home runs, but had 820 RBIs and scored 858 runs. The following season, even though the team hit 23 more home runs, the Tribe had only 760 RBIs and scored 790 runs.

One benefit of González's injury was the rise of Grady Sizemore. After appearing in 43 games in 2004, Sizemore became the Tribe's regular center fielder in 2005 and an All-Star from 2006 through 2008. He led the league in 2006 in runs scored and doubles and was superb defensively. Even though the Tribe might have made the post-season with a healthy González, Sizemore helped lead the Indians into the 2007 playoffs.

TREATMENT

Hamstring injuries are common in athletes who play sports that require powerful acceleration and deceleration. The hamstring muscles (see medical illustration, page 308) are some of the longest and fleshiest (thickest) muscles in the body, running down the back of the leg from the buttocks to below the knee. The muscles help flex the knee.

Hamstring injuries are classified as follows

- Grade 1—Mild muscle strain or pull
- Grade 2—Partial muscle tear
- Grade 3—Complete muscle tear

Hamstring tears usually occur at the muscle-tendon junction, an area that weakens with advancing age. This region is known to have decreased blood flow. The tears heal with significant scar tissue, which may ultimately shorten the muscle. A shortened hamstring muscle might reduce mobility and cause a limp.

Most hamstring injuries are treated with flexibility training, muscle strengthening, and physical therapy. Surgery is necessary when a complete upper attachment tear is involved. Operative management may also be required to control significant sciatic nerve symptoms from abundant scar tissue or when athletes are unable to regain their full range of motion or strength.

INCIDENTAL FINDING

The following is an excerpt from the Mitchell Report.

> Canadian Border Service Seizure of Steroids in Toronto, October 2001
>
> On the evening of October 4, 2001, Canadian Border Service officers working at Toronto's international airport discovered steroids, syringes, and clenbuterol in an unmarked duffel bag during an airport search of luggage that had been unloaded from the Cleveland Indians flight from Kansas City. Ted Walsh, the Indians equipment and clubhouse manager who was present during the search, recognized the bag as one that had been sent down to be included with the luggage by Cleveland outfielder Juan González when the Indians left Kansas City. On prior trips, González had included bags for members of his entourage with his own bags, and Walsh had the impression that this was the case with some of the bags he sent down to be packed for the Toronto flight....

Thereafter, Davidson, Haynes [a Canadian Border Service officer], and other officials watched the luggage as Joshue Perez, a member of Juan González's entourage, claimed the duffel bag. With Davidson present, Haynes and other officers took Perez to an anteroom, where he told them that the bag belonged to Angel ("Nao") Presinal, González's personal trainer, who would be arriving in Toronto on a later flight.

As soon as he arrived at the hotel, Presinal was detained by law enforcement officers. In an interview at the hotel, Presinal denied that the bag belonged to him and asserted that it belonged to, and had been packed by, González. Haynes and Toronto police officers then went to González's room to question him about the bag. Although he had been present for the interview of Presinal, Davidson was not invited to attend the interview of González. After that interview, Haynes reported that González had denied any knowledge about the bag's contents and claimed that he had sent it down to be included with the team's luggage at Presinal's request.

According to Davidson's account of the incident, during further questioning Presinal admitted that he had packed the steroids but claimed that he carried them for González, whom he helped to administer them. Davidson reported that Presinal also claimed to have assisted several other high-profile major league players in taking steroids. In our interview of him in 2007, Presinal denied that he made any such statements. He asserted that he has no knowledge of the involvement of any player in Major League Baseball with anabolic steroids or other performance enhancing substances. . . .

Rob Manfred [MLB's executive vice president for labor relations] told us that he did not believe a strong case could be made for "reasonable cause" testing of González because of conflicting statements by Presinal, González, and others about who the bag and steroids belonged to. Manfred nevertheless contacted Gene Orza of the Players Association about testing González, but Orza refused to agree in this instance. Manfred did not ask Orza for the Players Association's permission to interview González because he thought such an interview would be fruitless even if the Players Association agreed to it. (George J. Mitchell, "Report to the Commissioner of Baseball of an Independent Investigation into the Illegal Use of Steroids and Other Performance Enhancing Substances by Players in Major League Baseball," December 13, 2007)

Promises Not Kept

Travis Lee "Pronk" Hafner

Born: 1977
Cleveland Indians: 2003–07
Position: Designated Hitter / First Baseman
Jersey Number: 32 (2003); 48 (2004–12)

Grady Sizemore

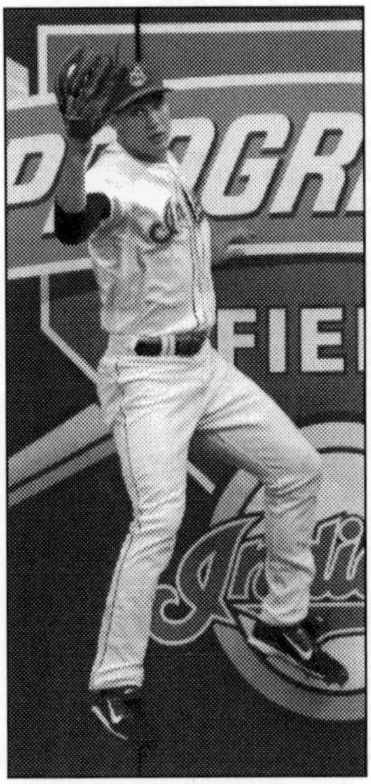

Born: 1982
Cleveland Indians: 2004–11
Position: Center Fielder
Jersey Number: 24

Grady Sizemore makes a catch at Progressive Field, 2008 (Courtesy *Akron Beacon Journal*)

Jacob Cauthen "Jake" Westbrook

Born: 1977
Cleveland Indians: 2001–10
Position: Pitcher
Jersey Number: 37

SYMPTOMS

Travis Lee Hafner was born and raised in North Dakota, attending a small high school in Sykeston. He went on to Cowley Junior College in Kansas and led the 1996 Tiger baseball team to a record of 51–13. The following year he helped the Tigers win the National Junior College Athletic Association National Championship. Hafner holds several school records, including RBIs in a season (82), RBIs in a career (161), doubles in a season (21), and doubles in a career (36). The Texas Rangers selected Hafner in the thirty-first round of the 1996 amateur draft.

After five seasons in the Texas minor league organization, the Indians traded for the slugger in December 2002 for Einar Díaz and Ryan Drese. Even though management would say otherwise, Hafner's acquisition was made to minimize the departure of Jim Thome, who had produced over 100 RBIs in all but one season of his Cleveland career.

Hafner came to Cleveland with his nickname—"Pronk," created by Hafner and his teammate Bill Selby, who was also a member of the Texas organization. A combination of "project" and "donkey," the final nickname was whittled down from "Pronky" and "El Pronko." After Pronk made his mark on the shores of Lake Erie, Malley's Chocolates of Cleveland manufactured a candy bar named after him.

Hafner made the opening day roster in 2003 and collected three hits. Unfortunately, he broke his left big toe against the Rangers on May 9. He was subsequently optioned back to Cleveland's Buffalo affiliate, where he sprained his wrist in early June, putting him on the disabled list. Hafner was called back up on July 12 and had respectable numbers for the remainder of the season. In 2004, Hafner showed the power the Indians had traded for, batting .311, with 28 home runs and 109 RBIs. The following year he batted .305, with 33 home runs and 108 RBIs. In 2006, Hafner belted out 42 home runs and led the league in on-base and slugging percentages, but was sidelined after breaking his hand in early September.

During the Tribe's 2007 season, Hafner signed a six-year extension worth $66 million. He had a solid season, but his statistics did not compare to the previous three seasons. In the postseason that year Hafner had two home runs, but batted only .186. In 2008, he suffered a shoulder injury and was limited to 57 games. He missed more games in 2009 and 2010 and ultimately had shoulder surgery. His home run totals in those three seasons dropped to 5, 16, and 13, respectively. He continued to battle injuries in 2011 and 2012 as he played out the remainder of his contract and signed on with the New York Yankees in 2013.

The Tribe could have been in the pennant race in 2008, but Hafner would have had to post near-career statistics. Unfortunately, instead of Pronk, Cleveland got Bronk, "bruised" and "zonked."

PATIENT HISTORY

"We have been tracking this guy [Hafner] since spring training. He's one of the most unique hitters in the minors. He hits for average and power, he gets on base, and he walks."
—Mark Shapiro, Cleveland general manager

"How big is Sykeston? I'd say about 180. It's really more of a wheat field. There were twenty-three people in my high school and eight in my graduating class."
—Travis Hafner

"I believe that Travis can become a consistent middle-of-the-order hitter. How much better he will get, only time will tell."
—Eric Wedge, Cleveland manager

SYMPTOMS

Grady Sizemore came to Cleveland in a 2002 deal that sent Bartolo Colon, the Tribe's ace at the time, and Tim Drew, a first-round pick in the 1997 amateur draft, to Montreal. Cleveland also received Cliff Lee, Lee Stevens, and Brandon Phillips, a rising shortstop who was the key player in the transaction. Mark Shapiro, Cleveland's general manager, wanted to rebuild the team and create another exciting contender to mirror the 1995–2001 years. Phillips spent less time in a Tribe uniform than Sizemore and the shortstop was traded to Cincinnati after an unheralded career in Cleveland. Lee Stevens played the remainder of the season for Cleveland and then retired from the game. Cliff Lee had several strong seasons for Cleveland, including a 22-win season in 2008 that led to the Cy Young award. He was traded to Philadelphia at the end of July 2009.

A star athlete, Sizemore had turned down a scholarship to play quarterback at the University of Washington before being drafted by the Montreal Expos in 2000. After playing for the Tribe's Akron and Columbus farm teams, Sizemore was brought up late in 2004. Although he was part of spring training for the Tribe in 2005, Sizemore was scheduled to return to Triple A, but when Juan González wasn't healthy enough for opening day, Sizemore was recalled. He played in 158 games, batted .289, and became a fan favorite. In March of 2006, Sizemore signed a six-year, $23.45 million deal. Sizemore was gifted with speed and power, leading the league in 2006 in runs scored and doubles. He was a three-time All-Star and won two Gold Gloves.

In 2007, he helped lead the Tribe to the postseason. He batted .375 in the American League Division Series against the Yankees, helping the Indians to a 3–1 series victory. His slump, where he batted .222, against Boston in the American League Championship Series contributed in part to a 4–3 loss to the Red Sox. Nonetheless, Sizemore came back strong the following year, belting a career-high 33 home runs and 90 RBIs. The future looked bright for the Tribe and the twenty-five-year-old Sizemore.

In early 2009, Sizemore couldn't participate in the World Baseball Classic due to a groin injury. After beginning the season, he suffered an elbow injury that limited him to the designated-hitter role for a time. The elbow injury didn't respond to treatment and the Cleveland outfielder was placed on the fifteen-day disabled list in early June. After being reactivated, the elbow injury continued to bother Sizemore and it eventually led to two surgeries in September—one for the elbow and another for a sports-related hernia.

After a seemingly successful spring training in 2010, with fans expecting Sizemore to put up 2008 numbers, Sizemore injured his knee sliding into first base in a May 16 game against the Orioles. Initially, the injury wasn't considered serious. However, Sizemore had to undergo microfracture surgery (see medical illustration, page 311) on June 4 to repair cartilage damage and was out for the season. In 2011, Sizemore appeared in 71 games, batting only .224. His surgically repaired knee was still causing him problems, forcing him to sit out games. During the off-season, Sizemore continued to rehab his knee, but suffered a back strain doing so. The strained back turned out to be a herniated disc and Sizemore underwent back surgery. His Tribe days were over.

PATIENT HISTORY

"And what you're starting to see now is maybe that once-in-a-decade convergence of effort, energy, athleticism, and baseball ability."
—Mark Shapiro, Cleveland general manager

"Grady is such a consistent player on both sides of the ball. Arguably, he is one of the best leadoff hitters in the game right now."
—Eric Wedge, Cleveland manager

> "Grady plays very aggressively, and sometimes injuries result. . . . It's difficult to ask someone to change the way he plays, because that could lead to other compensatory injuries."
> —Lonnie Soloff, Cleveland trainer

SYMPTOMS

Jake Westbrook, who had 110 strikeouts in 63 innings during his last season at Madison County High School (Georgia), was drafted in the first round of the 1996 draft by the Colorado Rockies. He was traded to Montreal in 1997, to the New York Yankees in 1999, and came to Cleveland with Zach Day and Ricky Ledee for outfielder David Justice. Westbrook was a solid starter for the Tribe, winning 15 or more games and pitching 200 or more innings from 2004–06.

Westbrook stumbled out of the gate in 2007 with a 1–2 record and 7.90 ERA before going on the disabled list with an abdominal strain; he was also experiencing elbow pain. Westbrook returned after the All-Star break and struggled. His record in early August was 3–7 with a 5.01 ERA. He found his form late in the season and won a crucial game against Oakland in September to put the Tribe back into the playoffs. Westbrook pitched against the Yankees in the American League Division Series and lost. He also started two games against the Boston Red Sox in the American League Championship Series, winning one and leaving the seventh and deciding game with the Tribe down by one run. Unfortunately, the bullpen couldn't keep the game close and the Indians lost 11–2. Although the Tribe defeat was disappointing, Westbrook remained prominent in the Indians' 2008 plans.

Westbrook experienced soreness in his right arm during spring training, but he was in the starting rotation on opening day in 2008. In late April, in a game against Minnesota, he suffered back pain due to an intercostal strain and was put on the disabled list. After returning against the White Sox, he experienced elbow pain (see medical illustration, page 303) and was put back on the disabled list. Westbrook was examined by the Angels' team doctor, Lewis Yocum, and had ulnar collateral ligament reconstruction or Tommy John surgery (named for Yankees' pitcher Tommy John, who first had the surgery in 1974). The blow to the pitching staff contributed to the Tribe's third place finish that year. Westbrook's rehabilitation forced him to sit out the entire 2009 season and after starting 6–7 with a 4.65 ERA in 2011, the hurler was traded to the St. Louis Cardinals as part of a three-team deal that brought Corey Kluber to the Indians. Westbrook posted good numbers in 2011 and 2012 for the Cardinals.

PATIENT HISTORY

> "Your dream is what gets you going. Your hard work is what gets you where you want to go. Your desire to be better is what helps you stay there."
> —Jake Westbrook

> "The kid has real good velocity and control."
> —Pat Daugherty, Colorado Rockies director of scouting

> "He's intelligent, a tough competitor. He has a quiet intensity about him that he channels in the right direction."
> —Eric Wedge, Cleveland manager

DIAGNOSIS

By acquiring Hafner, Sizemore, and Westbrook, Tribe brass was following the blueprint that had made the team the envy of most middle-market teams in the 1990s. They patiently rebuilt a team, became competitive, and made the postseason before losing to the New York Yankees and the Boston Red Sox. As they had done in the previous decade, the team decided to sign the three proven players, and fan favorites, as cornerstones of the franchise. Unfortunately, after they had signed contract extensions, injuries followed that put their playing careers in question. The Tribe was left without a center fielder, a power hitter, and a stopper in their rotation. Moreover, contract payments limited the moves the organization could make.

Almost immediately after the injury bug bit, the 2008, 2009, and 2010 seasons were disastrous on the field and at the gate. The Cy Young winners (C. C. Sabathia and Cliff Lee) were traded, a demoralizing blow to the fan base (Michael Brantley was the only starter the Tribe got from those deals.). Both players quickly won championships with other teams, which made the situation even more painful. The fans grew angry and eventually, apathetic. Victor Martinez, the team's popular catcher, was dispatched as well and the front office began unraveling the team. (Justin Masterson came as one of the players in the trade.) The Tribe's decline in paying customers and the financial obligations to the injured players hampered the team for years.

At their peak, Westbrook, Sizemore, and Hafner were the core of the team that came within a game of getting back to the World Series. In the 2007 postseason, Cleveland led the Red Sox three games to one with three chances to clinch the American League pennant, but watched as Boston made an unprecedented comeback, winning the series in seven games. Every Indians fan believed that the winner of the American League Championship Series would be the de facto World Series winner; the Colorado Rockies were viewed as an inferior opponent. Injuries kept cruel and unusual punishment coming to Tribe fans.

SECOND OPINION

During the Boston collapse in 2007, Hafner batted a paltry .148 and Sizemore fared little better (.222). The Indians as a team batted .254, compared to Boston's .318. The Tribe's pitchers posted a 6.82 ERA, with C. C. Sabathia chalking up a 10.45 ERA. Those numbers don't win series. The vacancy that really hurt the team was the loss of Cliff Lee, who was injured in spring training and never regained his form.

The 2007 team had some budding stars: Jhonny Peralta (twenty-five years old), Asdrubal Cabrerra (twenty years old), and Shin-Soo Chin (twenty-four years old). In 2008, Joe Borowski, who had 45 saves in 2007, saved only 6 games and the team totaled only 31 saves. Locking up a core of players to long-term deals was prudent, but even prudent franchises can't account for injuries.

TREATMENT

Tommy John surgery is a common term in baseball vernacular. The surgery refers to the reconstruction of the ulnar collateral ligament (UCL) in the elbow (see medical illustration, page 303). The UCL is a tough, strong triangular ligament, which gives the elbow support when an athlete is in the cocking position of throwing a baseball. The ligament undergoes a great amount of stress while pitching and, to a lesser extent, while throwing a football or serving a tennis ball. The UCL can be stretched, frayed, or torn. Pitchers with a torn UCL can no longer throw a ball with the same velocity they could prior to the injury.

Injuries to the ulnar collateral ligament (UCL) do not show up on X-rays and require an MRI to diagnose. If the ligament is torn, young athletes can play other positions or play other sports, such as football or wrestling. If they have promise as a pitcher, some athletes opt for Tommy John surgery, but it is not indicated for every hurler, considering the expense of the procedure and long recovery time (twelve to eighteen months).

The procedure is performed using a tendon from elsewhere in the body (usually from the forearm, hamstring, or knee) to create a new ligament. The surgery has a high success rate when performed by experienced surgeons. The surgery does not enable the pitcher to throw harder, as many parents and young players believe. The surgery does require intense physical therapy afterward, which improves the outcome. The one major risk of Tommy John surgery is damage to the ulnar nerve, which is close to the ligament.

Throwing mechanics are an important consideration as well. Rarely does the injury occur in young pitchers who are still growing. These pitchers usually stress and damage the growth plate on the inside of the elbow, a condition known as "Little League Elbow," for which surgery is not necessary.

INCIDENTAL FINDINGS

Tommy John had 288 lifetime wins. In a strange twist, he can trace his surgery fame to the Cleveland Indians. By the time he made his major league debut in 1963 for Cleveland, a season where he pitched 20.1 innings with a 2.21 ERA, he had already developed a sore arm pitching in the minors. Those were the days of playing through the pain and not complaining. From 1963 until 1974, John had around thirty five injections to quell the discomfort and swelling in his pitching arm. Eventually, he was pulled from a game because his arm was too weak and he couldn't get the ball to the plate.

John became a patient of Dr. Frank Jobe, the Dodgers' team doctor for over forty years. Jobe eventually received a special recognition award from the Baseball Hall of Fame. In part, he got his accolades for developing and refining a complex elbow procedure, the Tommy John surgery, which furthered the careers of hundreds of ballplayers. A 2013 study found that 124 active pitchers, about one-third of those in the majors, had undergone Tommy John surgery at some point in their careers. Dr. Jobe died in March 2014.

Cleveland Browns

1946–49 All American Football Conference
1950–95 National Football League
1999–present National Football League
Last Championship: 1964

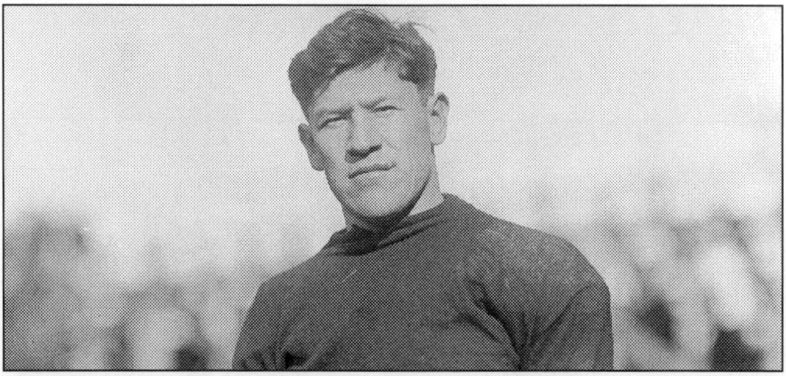

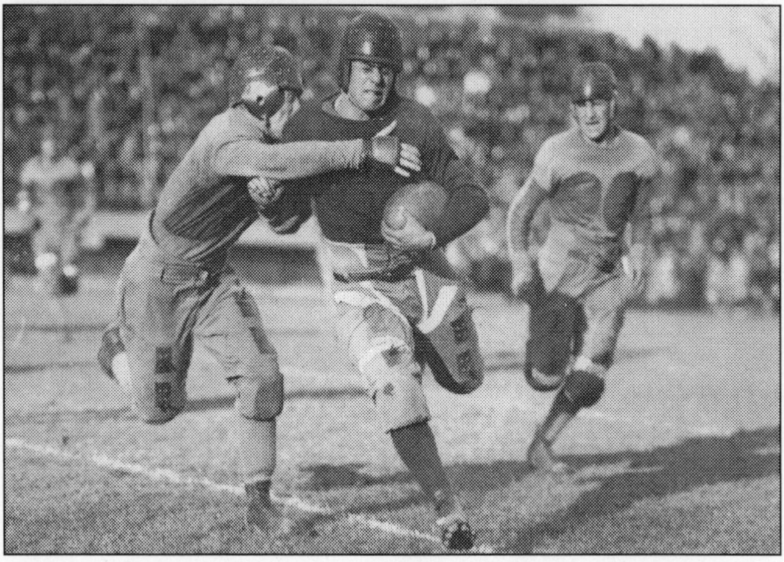

(Top) Jim Thorpe was a member of the Cleveland Tigers, 1920 (Library of Congress, Prints & Photographs Division, LC-DIG-hec-13257)

(Bottom) Action from a 1920s football game (Library of Congress, Prints & Photographs Division, LC-DIG-ds-03742)

The roots of football and great coaching can easily be traced back to Northeastern Ohio at the turn of the twentieth century. John Heisman coached at Oberlin College in 1892 and at Buchtel College (later the University of Akron) in 1893. Collegiate football aroused fan interest during the early 1900s. A 1913 game pitting Army against Navy drew 51,000 fans. (By comparison, the first Cleveland Browns game in 1946, drew 5,000 fans.)

Professional football got its start in the Canton/Massillon, Ohio, area. In 1920, the American Professional Football Association (APFA) was formed, with teams primarily from Illinois, Indiana, Ohio, and New York. Cleveland fielded an APFA team in 1920 (Tigers) and 1921 (Indians). In 1922, the APFA was renamed and became the National Football League (NFL). Cleveland was a NFL member in 1923 (Indians), 1924, 1925, and 1927 (Bulldogs), 1931 (Indians), 1937–42, 1944, and 1945 (Rams).

The Cleveland Browns took shape as part of the All-American Football Conference (AAFC) in 1946. The team was originally going to be called the Panthers, but another area team had already secured the name. After a contest in the local paper, the name "Browns" was chosen to honor the head coach Paul Brown. Brown wasn't too thrilled about having the team named after him, so a story floated around that the team was called the Browns because Joe Louis, the "Brown Bomber," was then the reigning heavy weight champion of the world.

Paul Brown built a pro football dynasty in Cleveland, posting a 167–53–8 record, four AAFC titles, three NFL crowns, and only one losing season in seventeen years. In the four seasons the Browns operated in the AAFC, they lost just four games. When the Browns joined the NFL in 1950, they continued their winning ways, playing in the next six championship games and winning the title in 1950, 1954, and 1955.

When Three Wasn't a Charm

Dante Bert Joseph "Gluefingers" Lavelli

Born: 1923 Died: 2009
Cleveland Browns: 1946–56
Position: Left End
Jersey Number: 56 (1946–51); 86 (1952–55)

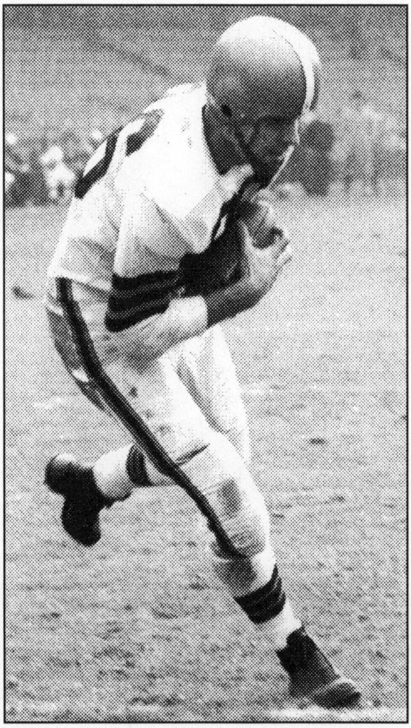

Dante Lavelli catches a touchdown against the Pittsburgh Steelers, 1952 (*The Cleveland Press* Collection, Cleveland State University, Fred Bottomer, photographer)

William Augustus "Dub" "Six-o-Clock" Jones

Born: 1924
Cleveland Browns: 1949–55
Position: Running Back / Flanker
Jersey Number: 86 (1949–51); 40 (1952–55)

Mac Curtis Speedie

Born: 1920 Died: 1993
Cleveland Browns: 1946–52
Position: Left End
Jersey Number: 58 (1946–51); 88 (1952)

SYMPTOMS

Although professional football had been played in Northeast Ohio for decades, the beginning of real fan interest in the game dates back to 1946, when the Cleveland Browns joined the All-American Football Conference under the leadership of Coach Paul Brown. The Browns won the league's championship from 1946–49 and then joined the NFL and won the championship in the team's first season in 1950. In 1951, the team again went to the championship game, but lost to the Los Angeles Rams. The Browns seemed poised to win the championship the following year, due in part to their trio of receivers, Dante "Glue Fingers" Lavelli, Dub "Six-o-Clock" Jones, and Mac Speedie.

Lavelli, who would go on to be enshrined in pro football's Hall of Fame, was All-AAFC and All-League twice, and after the Browns moved to the NFL, a starter in three of the first five Pro Bowl games. In the 1950 NFL Championship game, Lavelli caught 11 passes—then a record.

The lanky Jones was a running back/flanker for the Browns from 1948–55. He is one of three players (Ernie Nevers and Gale Sayers are the others) to score 6 touchdowns in a game and scored 29 touchdowns from 1950–52 to lead the league. After retiring, he was a Browns coach for several years.

Speedie played his entire career, from 1946–52, for the Browns. He earned various first-team All-League honors in every year except 1951. During his career, Speedie caught 349 passes for 5,602 yards (16.1 yards per catch) and made 33 touchdowns in just 86 regular season games.

In a September 1952 game against the Los Angeles Rams, Lavelli suffered a knee injury and was only be able to play in eight games during the rest of season. Without Lavelli, the Browns relied on Dub Jones and Mac Speedie to provide offense. Speedie led the league, catching 62 of Otto Graham's passes and Jones had 43 receptions. By the end of the season, Lavelli was healthy, but the last game against the New York Giants at the Polo Grounds put a damper on the

Browns' championship hopes. During the game, Dub Jones and Mac Speedie suffered leg injuries. With two weeks remaining before the Browns were to face the Lions at home in the championship game, the organization hoped the two stars would recover, creating a three-pronged attack that could ultimately undo the Lions' defense. Unfortunately, even though Speedie suited up for the Lions game, he never played a down, and Jones was on the sidelines, but in street clothes.

The Lions game was a rematch of an earlier contest in Detroit that season; the Lions had won, holding the Browns without a touchdown. This time, home field advantage was a factor in favor of the Browns. However, not having the trio of receivers in an offense that featured Otto Graham's strong arm led to a 17–7 loss. The Lions roared all the way back to Detroit.

PATIENT HISTORY

> "They talk about the bump-and-run nowadays. Heck, we had that with one difference. A defender didn't bump you, he knocked you down."
> —Dante Lavelli

> "Dub was a tall guy and a bit on the lean side. I remember Lou Rymkus [a Browns tackle from 1946–51] called him '6 o'clock' because he stood straight up and down."
> —Lou Groza, Football Hall of Famer

> "I would always watch Mac pick up things. He was tall and slender and really fast. He also had great moves. He could really fake out defensive backs."
> —Dante Lavelli

DIAGNOSIS

In the 1950s, the Cleveland Browns' roster was an embarrassment of riches. The team's talent, combined with the innovative coaching of Paul Brown, put the Browns several steps ahead of the league in football strategy and the acquisition of talent. The trio of Lavelli, Jones, and Speedie were unrivalled. The recurring injuries to the receiving corps, however, left the Browns vulnerable in the championship game and the Detroit Lions triumphed.

SECOND OPINION

The 1952 championship game was one the Browns should have easily won. The team outperformed the Lions, amassing 22 first downs to the Lions' 10 first downs; outgaining the Lions 227 yards to 199 yards; and throwing for 157 yard to the Lions 59 yards. However, as in all big games, turnovers played the deciding role. A pass that deflected off of one of the Browns' backs cost the team a touchdown at the beginning of the second half, and a Browns fumble on a punt by the Lions in the fourth quarter led to a Lions' field goal that sealed the victory.

A few years later, all three pass catchers would be gone from the Browns roster. Pete Brewster would replace Lavelli and have two Pro Bowl seasons. Preston Carpenter played right end for a few years. The biggest loss was probably at quarterback. After "Automatic" Otto Graham retired at the end of the 1955 season, the victories didn't come like they had.

TREATMENT

It was not uncommon during the 1950s and early 1960s for pro football players to have a full-time job away from the sport, since football salaries were not then the lucrative millions they are today. In most cases, players were only paid if they played. While precautions were taken, if a player could run, he undoubtedly would try to play.

The use of radiographs helped in determining the prognosis of certain bony injuries. However, without the availability of MRI and

CT scans or other more advanced testing techniques, extensive treatment of muscular, ligament, tendon, and cartilage injuries was limited.

Typical of the put-some-tape-on-it-and-go-back-in mentality of the early professional football era is an Otto Graham incident. In 1953, shortly before the end of the first half of an important Browns-49ers game, Otto Graham was knocked cold and carried off the field with a severe mouth injury. During half time, the team physician, Dr. Vic Ippolito and the trainer, Leo Murphy, began working on Graham. By the time the second half began Otto had somewhere between ten and fifteen stitches inside his mouth, which was almost swollen shut. Without protocols for treating concussions, Graham went back in the game, completed nine of ten passes, and the Browns won, 23–21.

INCIDENTAL FINDINGS

In the late 1920s, the problems of knee injuries were addressed in the *Canadian Medical Association Journal* (17, no. 11 (Nov. 1927): 1324–26).

> TREATMENT
>
> In all cases of simple traumatic synovitis, bruises, and direct hits, without evidence of rupture of a ligament, we have tried the following measures:
>
> A. Massage.
> B. Diathermic penetration [heat therapy using microwaves].
> C. Infrared rays.
> D. Static spark from a Wimshurst machine [developed in the 1800s by James Wimshurst to create static electricity].
>
> At present we start all the cases with the static spark for about five days, and find that the redness, swelling, and fluid disappear more rapidly under this line of treatment than any other. This is followed by massage and movements. All cases with lateral ligament injury we have treated as fractures, placing them in a plaster cast for not less than two months after the first swelling

has been reduced. The results are on the whole satisfactory, but the question of open operation on severe internal lateral ligament injury should be considered. Some of our cases we feel sure would have made a more rapid recovery if we had done an open operation with living suture repair.

CONCLUSIONS

1. Injury to the knee joint caused more permanent wastage in our team than all other accidents combined.
2. Of the severe injuries to the knee, rupture of the internal lateral ligament is the commonest, and should be treated as a fracture, and it is doubtful whether the patient should be permitted to play again.
3. The prognosis appears fairly good, but there are types that may call for open operation.
4. The injury appears to occur most often while on the defensive, when the knees are braced for resistance.

A Derailed Express

Ernest R. "The Elmira Express" Davis

Born: 1939 Died: 1963
Cleveland Browns: Drafted, never played
Position: Running Back
Jersey Number: 45

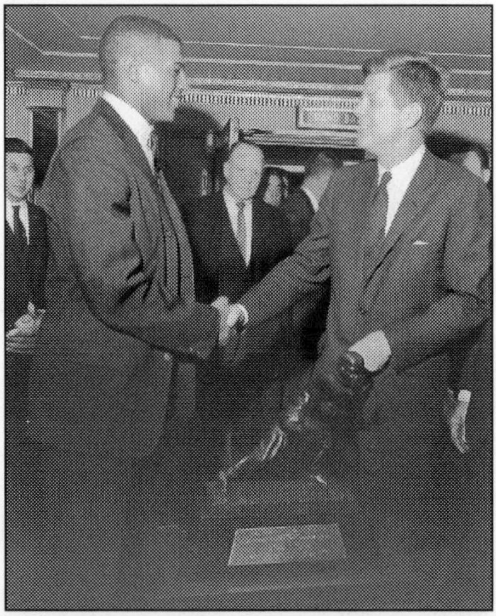

Heisman Trophy winner Ernie Davis greets President John F. Kennedy, 1961 (Cecil Stoughton, White House Photograph, John F. Kennedy Presidential Library and Museum, Boston)

SYMPTOMS

Ernie Davis was a high school receiver in Elmira, New York, but when he got to Syracuse University, he had filled out and was converted to running back. The Orangemen coach Ben Schwartswalder, who had previously had Jim Brown on his team, thought Davis was farther along in his sophomore year than Brown had been. Davis, a two-time All-American at six foot two and 210 pounds, won the Heisman Trophy in his senior year, the first African American to do so. Davis ended his college career at Syracuse with a seven yards per carry average and was coveted by teams in the established NFL and upstart AFL.

In 1961, the Browns finished in third place in the NFL's East Division, with a record of 8–5–1. The last time the Browns had won the

NFL crown was in 1955; the Browns played in the 1957 and 1958 championship games, but came out losers. The new owner Art Modell, who bought the team in 1961, wanted to bring a championship back to Cleveland. Modell was a hands-on guy, unlike many of the Browns' former owners, which impacted his relationship with Paul Brown. Brown was used to having complete player personnel authority.

Prior to the 1962 NFL Draft, Coach Brown—without consulting Modell—orchestrated a deal with the Redskins, who drafted Ernie Davis with the first pick and then traded Davis to the Browns for Bobby Mitchell and the rights to rookie Leroy Jackson, the Browns' first-round pick. Even though Jim Brown thought Mitchell was the best breakaway back in the league, and Brown and Mitchell made a spectacular backfield, Paul Brown and others in the organization envisioned a new Browns dynasty with the tandem of Brown and Davis leading the way. The Browns signed Davis to a three-year, no-cut, no-trade $65,000 contract with a $15,000 signing bonus, but friction now existed between Jim Brown, Art Modell, and Paul Brown.

Until the tradition was discontinued after 1976, teams of college All-Stars played against the NFL champions prior to the regular season. Ernie Davis was to play in the 1962 contest. The All-Stars began practice in mid-July for the August 3 game in Chicago. A few days before the contest, Davis was hospitalized with what was thought to be the mumps or mononucleosis, but both were ruled out. A few weeks prior to the incident, Davis had wisdom teeth removed and checked into an Evanston hospital because postsurgery bleeding couldn't be stopped. Eventually, Davis was diagnosed with a blood disorder. Davis went through a series of tests in Cleveland and was transferred to the National Institutes of Health in Maryland for further evaluation. Ultimately, Davis was told he had acute monocytic leukemia (a type of acute myeloid leukemia).

Over the next several months, Davis had periods of weight loss and extreme fatigue, but he also experienced periods of remission, feeling strong and pain-free. Davis practiced when healthy and was determined to make a comeback. Even though the Browns held out hope that Davis could overcome the disease and the organization did all they could to help the ailing star, he lost his battle in May 1963 and died at the age of twenty-three. If fans felt that a curse hung over the Browns, two other 1963 incidents confirmed the belief. Twenty-five-year-old starting safety Don Fleming, who seemed destined to become an All-Pro, was electrocuted while working in Florida during the off-season. Prior to Davis's death, Tom Bloom, a Browns draftee out of Purdue University, had died in a winter car accident.

In 1964, after Paul Brown was fired and replaced by Blanton Collier, the Browns would win the NFL Championship, but the death of Davis, the loss of Mitchell, and the early retirement of Jim Brown after the 1965 season altered the future of the Browns for decades.

PATIENT HISTORY

> "The thing I recall most vividly is the fact that you never heard this guy [Davis] complain about the illness. Never heard him say he got a tough break."
> —John Wooten, Browns guard

> "He'd probably be living today if he were stricken with the same illness, with all the medications available now."
> —Art Modell, Cleveland Browns owner

> "When I look back, I can't call myself unlucky. My twenty-third birthday was December 14. In these years, I have had more than most people get in a lifetime."
> —Ernie Davis

DIAGNOSIS

Ernie Davis's story might be the most heart-wrenching story that Cleveland sports fans have endured. The Browns wanted to bring Davis to Cleveland for all the right reasons. He was a great athlete, and by every account, a wonderful human being. If all was fair in the world of sports, he would have been running the football, scoring touchdowns, and helping the team win championships well into the 1970s. He might have ended up in the Pro Football Hall of Fame. Instead, fans were left with only a vision of the "dream backfield."

In the meantime, Bobby Mitchell had a great second half of his career in Washington and ended up in the Pro Football Hall of Fame. Cleveland Browns owner Art Modell and head coach Paul Brown were already at odds, but the death of Ernie Davis seemed to push them further apart. The loss was much more devastating than anything that could ever occur on the field.

SECOND OPINION

Ernie Davis would undoubtedly have helped the Browns, especially after the retirement of Jim Brown. Still, the 1964 draft brought two Hall of Famers to the club—Paul Warfield and Leroy Kelly. In the last Jim Brown year, the Browns lost to the Packers in the 1965 championship game. The following year, they missed the postseason. In 1967, the Browns were crushed by the Dallas Cowboys 52–14 in the division playoff game. The next year, the team rebounded and beat the Cowboys in the division playoff game, but lost to the Colts in the conference championship game, 34–0.

Art Modell's relationship with both Paul Brown and Jim Brown didn't help the situation. However, the defense was not up to the task during the postseason and perhaps for any number of reasons, the Browns didn't play well enough in the big games.

TREATMENT

Leukemia is a cancer of the blood or the bone marrow where blood cells are formed. The disease causes an abnormal increase in the number of white blood cells. There are four major types of leukemia:

Acute lymphocytic leukemia (ALL). Patients with ALL have too many immature white blood cells in their bone marrow. ALL is the most common childhood cancer, but 95 percent of children with ALL attain remission.

Acute myeloid leukemia (AML). AML prevents the body from making normal red blood cells, white blood cells, and platelets. The five-year survival rate for AML is about 25 percent.

Chronic lymphocytic leukemia (CLL). CLL is the most common form of adult leukemia. CLL leads to overproduction of certain white blood cells. The average five-year survival rate for someone with CLL is between 50 percent and 80 percent.

Chronic myeloid leukemia (CML). CML is a rare leukemia resulting from a change in a person's DNA. The five-year survival rate for CML has nearly doubled from 31 percent for people diagnosed between 1990 and 1992 to 59 percent for those diagnosed between 2003 and 2009.

The signs and symptoms of leukemia include increased bruising or bleeding excessively because of a lack of blood platelets. Patients may become pale and short of breath, secondary to anemia. Infections are more common in leukemia patients because the white blood cells, which fight infection, do not work normally. Other symptoms include fevers, chills, night sweats, and fatigue. Patients often experience weight loss. Leukemia is usually diagnosed through blood tests or a bone marrow biopsy.

Treatment of leukemia may include chemotherapy, radiation, or a bone marrow transplant. The prognosis for patients with leukemia changed dramatically through the 1960s and 1970s. Since then, the survival rate has improved.

INCIDENTAL FINDINGS

From 1934 until 1976, the best collegiate football players battled the NFL champions annually each August in Chicago. Ernie Davis was supposed to play against the Green Bay Packers in the 1962 contest, which the Packers won 42–20. The Cleveland Browns played against the College All-Stars in 1951, 1955, 1956, and 1965. They won three times, but lost to the collegians in 1955 by a score of 30–27. Ralph Guglielmi, a quarterback from Notre Dame, was named the 1955 MVP.

Double-teamed by the Philadelphia Turf

Jerry Martin Sherk

Born: 1948
Cleveland Browns: 1970–81
Position: Defensive Lineman
Jersey Number: 72

SYMPTOMS

Jerry Sherk joined the Cleveland Browns in 1970 after attending Oklahoma State University. Sherk was an All-Big-Eight football star and an All-American wrestler before being selected in the second round (forty-seventh overall) of the NFL Draft. (Mike Phipps, a quarterback from Purdue University, was chosen in the first round by the Browns and third overall.) Sherk's duel-athletic talent was perfect for a NFL defensive lineman.

Sherk's first career start was against the New York Jets in the inaugural *Monday Night Football* telecast. Watched by millions, Sherk was schooled all night long by Jets right guard Randy Rasmussen. Howard Cosell let listeners know, especially in the second half, that Sherk was being manhandled. The Browns' defensive tackle, however, got back up and became a four-time Pro Bowl selection. He was chosen as the top defensive linemen in 1975 and was voted the Browns MVP in 1974 and 1975 by his teammates.

The football career of the Browns' premier defensive lineman changed during a 1977 exhibition game against the Green Bay Packers. Sherk stretched ligaments in his left knee and he was out of action for several weeks, starting only six games. When he did play, he had lost some quickness—a vital part of his skill set. During the final game of the season against Seattle, Sherk injured his right knee, requiring off-season surgery.

By 1979, Cleveland fans had gone through five consecutive losing seasons. The Browns, however, seemed poised to change the trend. Jerry Sherk was healthy again after a subpar 1978 campaign. The team got out of the gate fast, winning their first four contests. After three consecutive losses, they bounced back with two wins and faced the Philadelphia Eagles. On that November day, an infected boil on Sherk's arm was scraped off by the artificial turf, resulting in a staph infection. Sherk had 12 sacks in 10 games, helping an improving defense and allowing the Brian Sipe-led offense to put up points and win games. Without Sherk, the team went 2–4 over the last six games and missed the playoffs by only one game. A healthy Sherk could have propelled the team into the postseason.

Sherk almost lost his life when the staph infection entered his bloodstream, causing a septic infection. Hospitalized for six weeks, he dropped over fifty pounds. Sherk was only able to return for one game in 1980 and played sparingly as a pass-rush specialist during the 1981 season before retiring. His possible Hall of Fame career was ended by the turf in the city of not-so-brotherly love.

PATIENT HISTORY

"What Jerry accomplished on the field are achievements that made him the best tackle in Browns' history."
—Art Modell, Cleveland Browns owner

"[During my early years] I was feeling my way and learning the position. The middle four years, I had mastered the position and felt I could dominate. The last three years, I knew what to do but my body couldn't do it."
—Jerry Sherk

"He came to the meeting after the Philadelphia game and his leg swelled so big they couldn't get his pant leg off."
—Sam Rutigliano, Browns coach

DIAGNOSIS

Jerry Sherk's injury epitomizes how fate and medical mishaps derailed the Browns' chance to get to a Super Bowl. The 1970 Browns were a good team, but hardly as strong as the title contenders of 1960s and the "Team of Champions" of the 1950s. By the middle of the decade, the Browns were in a full-fledged collapse, posting a 4–10 record in 1974 and going 3–11 in 1975, only the second and third losing seasons in the thirty-year history of the franchise.

The Browns began to rebound in 1978 under new coach Sam Rutigliano, finishing at 8–8, and the following year the team posted a 9–7 record. In 1980, the Browns, known that year as the "Kardiac Kids" (13 of their 16 games were decided in the last two minutes) returned to the playoffs and looked like a Super Bowl contender. Unfortunately, Sherk wasn't available to bolster the defensive line. Small differences can separate teams and trophies. Sherk was a star when the team was down, and he was down when the Browns needed him most.

SECOND OPINION

When Sherk played ten games in 1979, the Browns defense was ranked twentieth overall. The following year, the defense moved up to twelfth. The Sipe-led 1980 offense was eighth in the NFL, winning games by an average margin of 2.9 points. Cleveland was not favored in their 1980 playoff game against Oakland. The weather didn't help, with a game-time wind chill of -20 degrees.

The frozen conditions led to seven turnovers, four by the Browns. On defense, the Browns held Oakland to 208 total yards. Unfortunately, the final Browns turnover, which came as they were driving for a touchdown rather than taking a chance on a field goal, ended their season.

The following year, the team fell back to 5–11 and the last-minute heroics vanished. However, the 1979 and 1980 drafts hadn't helped.

Willis Adams, a wide receiver out of Houston, was the Browns' top pick in 1979 and Charles White was chosen as the number one pick in 1980. Neither became stars.

TREATMENT

Bacteria called staphylococcus aureus cause most staph infections in the body. In Greek, the term translates to "a bunch of grapes," which is what a staph infection looks like under a microscope. These bacteria can normally be found on the skin and in the noses of 25–30 percent of healthy adults. In the majority of cases, the immune system helps prevent the bacteria from causing infection. Damage to the skin, such as a scrape or a cut, allows staph to get past the first line of defense.

Staph infections initially can present as a boil, an infected hair follicle, or an abscess (collection of pus under the skin), but can progress to impetigo (crusting of the skin) or cellulitis (an infection deeper into the connective tissue between muscle and skin). At this later stage, the infection is usually accompanied by redness, warmth, and systemic symptoms (fever, chills, low blood pressure, etc.).

If the infection continues untreated or the body's defense system is overwhelmed, the infection can quickly spread to the bloodstream, resulting in septic shock (a significant life-threatening drop in blood pressure) or spread to the bones (osteomyelitis), joints (septic arthritis), heart (endocarditis), and lungs (pneumonia). To avoid these complications, early diagnosis and antibiotic treatment is crucial. Although widespread cases of staph infection are rare, 20–40 percent of cases that spread to the bloodstream result in death.

In the 1980s, a strain of staph bacteria developed that did not respond to simple penicillin-like antibiotic treatments. The strain occurred almost exclusively in hospitals with patients that had severely compromised immune systems. The hospital-acquired bacteria were much more difficult to treat and it was believed that the "super bug" developed because of the overuse of strong antibiotics.

In the 1990s, the bacteria started to cause infections outside of hospitals and nursing homes and became known as community-acquired MRSA (methicillin-resistant staphylococcus aureus). Some of the most common settings for MRSA are sports locker rooms, training rooms, and artificial turf. Frequent skin abrasions and the sharing of personal items (towels, shavers, water bottles, etc.) in these settings promote bacteria growth. The MRSA strain is more resistant to treatment and, therefore, is more likely to cause systemic symptoms and to spread to the bloodstream. MRSA also may develop "flesh-eating" complications which may lead to amputations and death.

INCIDENTAL FINDINGS

Jerry Sherk was an outstanding wrestler at Oklahoma State University (OSU). He won the Big Eight Conference heavyweight championship in 1970. OSU has been and continues to be a NCAA wrestling powerhouse. Sherk attributes wrestling with making him more agile and quicker on the gridiron.

Sherk's linemate Walter Johnson tried his hand at professional wrestling during the Johnny Powers era in Cleveland. Unfortunately, Johnson couldn't translate his football skills to the mat. In the spring of 1969, Powers teamed up with Johnson to take on the Love Brothers, a tandem that donned psychedelic pants and beads. In a controversial decision, the Love Brothers took two out of three falls and won the match. Johnson never got to use his submission moves—the flying tackle or bear hug.

Storming into Cleveland

Lyle Martin Alzado

Born: 1949 Died: 1992
Cleveland Browns: 1979–81
Position: Defensive Lineman
Jersey Number: 77

SYMPTOMS

In 1978, the Cleveland Browns finished with a record of 8–8, but their defense was twenty-fifth in the league. When the opportunity to bolster the defensive line arose in 1979, the Browns traded two future draft picks (the 1980 second-round and 1981 third-round picks) for Denver star Lyle Alzado, who was considered one of the top defensive linemen in the league. According to various reports, Alzado was to get $220,000 per year, which was topped only by Brain Sipe's salary of $300,000.

Alzado was a character to say the least; he fought in an exhibition bout against Muhammad Ali, he made home exercise tapes for men, and he owned a disco during his time in Denver. The defensive lineman had been accused of wild mood swings and abuse by an ex-wife; in one game he ripped someone's helmet off and threw it at an offensive lineman (which resulted in the Alzado rule—"the removal of another player's helmet shall result in an ejection and possible fine"). In 1983, when Alzado was playing for the Raiders in the Super Bowl, the lineman threatened to behead Redskins quarterback Joe Theismann.

Alzado eventually attributed much of his erratic behavior to steroid use that began at Yankton College in South Dakota. Alzado also had a very tough childhood in the New York City area, dealing with a father who was an alcoholic and prone to violence. In high school, Alzado had many run-ins with the law and wasn't averse to fighting during football contests.

The former Denver Bronco had three good years with the Browns, including the 1980 "Kardiac Kids" season. That year the Browns' playoffs ended with the interception of a Brian Sipe pass by Raiders' Mike Davis on the infamous "Red Right 88" play. Alzado led the Browns in sacks during two of his three seasons; he was All-AFC in 1979 and All-Pro in 1980. During the 1980 season, Alzado's presence helped the defense rank twelfth in the league. However, the 1981 Browns finished a dismal 5–11.

Prompted by the team's poor performance, the Browns went on a youth movement and traded draft picks (first round in 1983, second round in 1984, and third round in 1985) for Tom Cousineau, the Buffalo Bill's first pick in the 1979 draft, who chose to play in Canada. Cousineau had starred locally at St. Edward High School and The Ohio State University. With Cousineau on board, the Browns couldn't pay Alzado the amount he wanted. Moreover, Alzado had injured himself during the previous training camp and was seeing a psychiatrist "for extreme mental pressure." Alzado was traded to the Oakland Raiders for an eighth-round draft pick and won a Super Bowl with the silver and black.

Alzado died of a brain tumor in 1992 at the age of forty-three. He attributed the condition to years of steroid use, but medical experts differed on the cause of Alzado's cancer. By the time of his death, he was frail and barely able to walk.

PATIENT HISTORY

> "I'd threaten their kids, their family, tell a guy he was ugly and that he'd be dead by the end of the game."
> —Lyle Alzado

> "You get a guy [Alzado] like that once in a while. His intensity rubs off on the other players. He's moody, he has his ups and downs, but let him go sit in a corner, I don't care. I know the next morning he'll be jumping all over the place."
> —Red Miller, Broncos head coach

"Alzado will be the first of a lot of big names to come down with cancers."
—Dr. Forest Tennant, the NFL's drug adviser, 1986–1990

DIAGNOSIS

Lyle Alzado was a fan favorite during his three years in the brown and orange, especially during the memorable "Kardiac Kids" season. He was a wild man on the field, but his behavior off the field became a problem, too. Stories surfaced about him, including that he threw a chair at a newspaper reporter and that he assaulted a female police officer after being stopped for a traffic violation. His time in Cleveland was turbulent. His story, perhaps more than any other athlete's, might have had the most impact on the NFL's tough stance against steroids in the early 1990s.

SECOND OPINION

The Browns gave up three picks (second- and fifth-round choices in 1980; third-round choice in 1981) to Denver to land Alzado. He started 46 games in his three-year career with Cleveland. With one of their picks, Denver chose Rulon Jones, who ended up having a stellar career with the team. The Cleveland defense was twenty-fourth, twenty-third, and twenty-third in Alzado's three years. The offense was ninth, eighth, and twenty-fourth in points scored. The difference in 1980, which propelled the team to the playoffs, was the fact that the defense was twelfth in points allowed. Unfortunately, the Alzado-led defense never rose to championship caliber.

TREATMENT

"'Roid rage" is a term given to the hostile, aggressive actions that sometimes occur in people who abuse anabolic steroids. These people can become highly irritable and at times violent. There have been several accounts of murders, brutal attacks, and suicides linked to steroid abuse. People abusing steroids may become paranoid and delusional; they are also prone to severe mood swings. Research indicates that those most vulnerable to developing steroid abuse are those with a prior history of aggressive behavior. Because of the adverse side effects of steroid abuse cessation (including an increased risk of depression and suicide), steroid addiction can be difficult to overcome without the help of trained medical professionals.

INCIDENTAL FINDINGS

Yankton College was founded in 1881 and closed its doors in 1984. In 1889, the college started its football program and became known as the Greyhounds. Primarily playing regional contests, the Yankton eleven had early success playing opponents like Huron College, the South Dakota School of Mines, and Dakota Wesleyan.

At Yankton, Lyle Alzado was named All Tri-state Intercollegiate Athletic Conference twice and a Little All-American. Still, he might not have made it to the NFL without a little luck. Stan Jones, a coach for the Denver Broncos, was on a scouting trip in Montana in 1971 when his car broke down. With time on his hands, he visited Montana Tech University and saw a film of the 1970 Copper Bowl; the Tech Orediggers had defeated Yankton. One player, an undersized defensive lineman who was in on every play, stood out on the Yankton team. The Denver coach persuaded the Broncos to select the player in the fourth round of that year's draft. Lyle Alzado, the Copper Bowl's Most Valuable Player, went to Denver and became part of the famed "Orange Crush."

The Closeness of Almost Being

Bernard Joseph "Bernie" "The Stork" Kosar Jr.

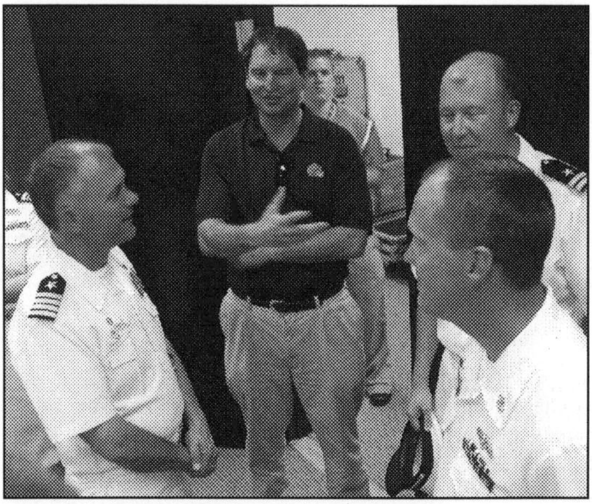

Born: 1963
Cleveland Browns: 1985–93
Position: Quarterback
Jersey Number: 19

Bernie Kosar welcomes US Navy sailors before a Browns and Chicago Bears game during Navy Week in Cleveland, Ohio, 2006 (Courtesy National Archives, Jason J. Perry, photographer)

SYMPTOMS

The 1984 Browns featured a quarterback named Paul McDonald who threw for 14 touchdowns and 23 interceptions. The team finished 5–11 in the first post-Brian-Sipe season. McDonald, out of USC, didn't seem to be the answer for the organization, and owner Art Modell was looking to beef up the offensive productivity by finding a college star to put behind center in Cleveland.

Bernie Kosar had been a phenomenal quarterback for Boardman High School in Youngstown, Ohio. In his senior year, he was a *Parade* magazine All-American. Long before LeBron James, Kosar took his talents to South Beach, not to the Heat, but to the Hurricanes. As a redshirt freshman in 1983, he led the Hurricanes to a 12–1 record and the school's first national championship. Kosar still holds several records at Miami, including the career completion percentage mark.

Kosar finished his college degree in three years and passed up two additional seasons of college eligibility to enter the 1985 supplemental draft. Cleveland outmaneuvered the Minnesota Vikings by making a deal with the Buffalo Bills to acquire the rights to Kosar. The Browns gave up their first-round picks in the 1985 and 1986 drafts, a 1985 third-rounder, and a 1986 sixth-rounder. Kosar was thrilled to come back home and hoped to lead the Browns to a Super Bowl.

In his inaugural season with the team, Kosar was thrust into the starter's role in early October after quarterback Gary Danielson injured his shoulder against the New England Patriots. Relying heavily on the rushing of Kevin Mack and Earnest Byner for the remainder of the regular season, the Browns finished 8–8 and made the playoffs. Although the 12–4 Miami Dolphins defeated the team, Bernie Kosar looked like a quarterback who could bring victories to the shores of Lake Erie.

The following two years, 1986 and 1987, were both memorable and devastating for the Browns and Kosar. Under the leadership of Kosar, the 1986 Browns finished with a regular season record of 12–5, defeated the New York Jets in the division championship game (where Kosar threw for almost 500 yards), and made it to the conference championship game to face the Denver Broncos. In remarkable contest, noted for "The Drive," John Elway led his team to a last-second touchdown to tie the score. The Broncos prevailed in overtime on a Rich Karlis field goal, which some Browns' fans contend—to this day—was wide left.

Undaunted by the outcome, the 1987 Browns made it back to the conference championship game against the Broncos in Denver. After a dismal start to the contest, during which Denver jumped to a 21–3 lead, Kosar choreographed a stunning comeback. With little time left on the clock, the Browns were inside the Denver ten-yard line and were in a position to tie the game. Misfortune struck again; Earnest Byner took a hand-off from Kosar and headed into the end zone, but lost the ball and Denver recovered "The Fumble." Denver sent Cleveland home again.

The Cleveland Browns were favored to make it to the 1988 Super Bowl because Kosar had proven he could shine in big games. Unfortunately, injuries got in the way. In August, Kosar bruised the thumb on his throwing hand during a preseason practice. Playing against the Kansas City Chiefs in September, Kosar strained a ligament in his right elbow and was sidelined until October 23. The final blow to Kosar's season came against the Dolphins in early December, when he sprained the medial collateral ligament in his knee. He missed the playoff game against Oakland, a Browns 24–23 loss.

In the 1989 season, the Browns lost to Denver in the conference championship game for the third time in four years. Kosar had a miserable game, completing only 19 of 44 attempts and throwing 3 interceptions. His play was affected by an index finger injury suffered during a playoff win against the Buffalo Bills, which forced Kosar to wear a splint on his throwing hand during the first half in Denver. He had also developed a staph infection in his right arm. His playoff game performance mirrored his regular season performance. In an October contest, Kosar threw a career high 4 interceptions and had a career low completion percentage of 36.5. (Of course, he was getting sacked more often, too—34 times in 1989, 37 times in 1990, and 41 times in 1991.)

Kosar started 13 games in 1990 and the Browns' record was a dismal 3–13. He started all 16 games the following year under new coach Bill Belichick, but the team sputtered to a 6–10 finish. Kosar suffered a hairline fracture of his ankle against the Dolphins in the second game of the 1992 season and didn't return until November 29. In the final game against the Steelers, a Cleveland loss, Kosar fractured his right ankle and required surgery.

Belichick decided that Kosar, often injured and with "diminishing skills," was not the answer and the team released Kosar in 1993. The former Cleveland quarterback signed with Dallas and won a Super Bowl that year as a backup to Troy Aikman. Kosar finished his career as a Miami Dolphin at age thirty-three in 1996.

Kosar was a fan favorite. When healthy, he was as skilled as any quarterback in the league. His performances in the first two championship games against Denver were outstanding, but the images

Cleveland Browns fans will never forget are the celebrations of the Broncos after Cleveland's heartbreaking losses.

PATIENT HISTORY

"He [Kosar] has an overall feel for things out there. The little things, like when to look off his primary receiver, how long to stay with another receiver, feeling a blitz, feeling when the blitz is a fake. He plays football like Isiah Thomas plays basketball. He knows where everyone is at all times."
—Gary Danielson, Browns' quarterback

"He [Kosar] wasn't afraid to pull the trigger. That made him special. His arm was sub-special, but everything else was special."
—Howard Schnellenberger, Kosar's college coach

"Nobody in the history of football looked so far opposite of where the ball was going."
—Jerry Glanville, Houston Oilers' coach

DIAGNOSIS

Browns fans will always remember Bernie Kosar fondly because he left college early and worked through many NFL challenges to join the team. He led the Browns to the brink of the Super Bowl, with three conference championship appearances in his first five seasons as the team's quarterback. Kosar continued to keep the dream alive as he battled through several injuries. The finger injury, which he suffered in the playoffs, was one of the most ill-timed of his career. The injury contributed to the trilogy of the Cleveland versus Denver sports tragedies known as "The Drive," "The Fumble," and "The Finger."

Kosar took the high road in his battles with Bill Belichick. He maintained his allegiance to the Cleveland Browns and the city throughout his football career and into retirement. For that reason, the gangly quarterback will always be a favorite son to the city's sports fans.

SECOND OPINION

Scooter Molander was part of the 1989 Browns, a small part. Molander was a quarterback that the team brought to training camp and then waived before the season started. The Colorado State alum was then signed to the Kansas City Chiefs developmental squad. The Browns went into the season with Bernie Kosar as their starter and Mike Pagel as his backup.

From 1986 through 1989, Pagel appeared in 10 games and started 4 times. In 1990, he threw the ball 14 times and completed 5 passes. The following year, he would start 3 games and lose them all. The Browns undoubtedly did not have full confidence in his abilities.

On January 14, 1990, the Browns were one step away from getting to the Super Bowl. The Denver Broncos were once again the team that stood in the way at Mile High. The week before, in a win against Buffalo, Kosar had smashed his hand against a Bills' shoulder pad and probably partially tore a ligament in his index finger. He also was suffering from a slightly dislocated shoulder, a bruised elbow, and a staph infection. Half a Kosar seemed better than a full Pagel, and Kosar played with two injured fingers, which led to a subpar performance and a trip home rather than to New Orleans.

Although Kosar was still in his prime, his injuries were mounting. The Browns might have been wise to draft a quarterback when they had a chance to do so. Pittsburgh chose Neil O'Donnell in the third round of the 1990 draft. The Browns picked a quarterback in that draft, too. With the 296th pick, they chose Clemente Gordon from Grambling.

TREATMENT

A "jammed finger" in sports usually involves one of four types of injuries:

- Ligament sprain. The middle joint of the finger is like a three-sided box and when the finger is jammed the ligament tears (see medical illustration, page 307). This "sprain," like an ankle sprain, needs a splint and rest. Rehabilitation is needed to regain a full range of motion and strength. A ligament injury is the most common result of a jammed finger.
- Extensor tendon rupture. The tendon that straightens the finger pulls off the bone in this injury. Known as "Mallet finger" or "baseball finger," this injury can be treated with a splint that keeps the finger fully straight for eight weeks. If it is not treated correctly, the end of the finger droops, causing a "drop finger." People can still play sports and work effectively with drop finger but they can't straighten the digit completely.
- Flexor tendon injury. The tendon that bends the finger is pulled off the bone. Known as "jersey finger" (a finger gets caught and twisted in an opponent's jersey), the injury greatly inhibits mobility. Surgery is required.
- Fracture with or without dislocation. A break in one of the bones of the finger, which requires the finger to be immobilized with a splint or cast. Surgery may be required if the finger does not heal itself. Unlike the other three types of injuries, an X-ray can help in diagnosis.

A 2008 study in the *American Journal of Sports Medicine* (36, no. 10, October 2008) investigated hand injuries suffer by NFL players. Dislocations and fractures were the most common injuries to the fingers; sprains to the fingers were also likely. Defensive secondary positions (safeties and cornerbacks) sustained 231 hand injuries (17 percent of all injuries), followed by offensive linemen (214 injuries, 16 percent of all injuries), defensive linemen (192 injuries, 14 percent of all injuries), and wide receivers (172 injuries, 12 percent of all injuries). The fewest injuries occurred in tight ends, with 5 percent of the total injuries. Quarterbacks sustained 93 injuries (7 percent of all injuries) to the hand, which was the second lowest total of any position.

INCIDENTAL FINDINGS

Bernie Kosar might have just been in the wrong place at the right time. The back-to-back stunners against the Broncos in the playoffs were tragic for Cleveland fans. Kosar had faced even more setbacks; during his junior year at Boardman High School, after the team started out at 6–0 and was a sure lock for the high school playoffs, a teacher's strike ended the season. Doug Flutie threw a dagger into the University of Miami's heart and a Hail Mary into the arms of Gerard Phelan after Kosar had seemingly won the game for the Hurricanes, driving his team ninety yards for a go-ahead touchdown and leaving only twenty-eight seconds on the clock. And of course, "The Fumble" came on a play called "13 Trap."

Kosar's postfootball life has included several bizarre incidents, a messy divorce, and DUI charges. The former Browns quarterback has also faced financial troubles and lost his job as a Browns analyst. Kosar has been forthcoming about the fact that hits sustained as a player might have caused years of headaches, insomnia, slurred speech, and persistent ringing in his ears. All that bad karma doesn't seem right for an altar boy from St. Mary's.

A Glimpse and Gone

Donald Lavert "Don" Rogers

Born: 1962 Death: 1986
Cleveland Browns: 1984–85
Position: Defensive Back
Jersey Number: 20

SYMPTOMS

The Browns were busy prior to the 1984 season. To cement the defensive backfield, the Browns selected Don Rogers out of UCLA with their first-round pick (eighteenth overall) of the NFL Draft. Rogers was signed to five one-year contracts worth a reported $1.7 million. The Browns selected Brian Brennan in the fourth round and Ernest Byner in the tenth round of the draft. In the supplemental draft, the Browns picked up Kevin Mack. The team also signed Frank Minnifield out of the USFL. Minnifield would be paired with Hanford Dixon to create one of the best sets of cornerbacks in the league.

The six-foot-one, 206-pound Rogers grew up in Sacramento, California, and went on to play at UCLA. In four seasons, the Bruins safety averaged over 100 tackles per season and was named the MVP in the 1982 Rose Bowl. In 1984, Rogers started 14 games for the Browns, missing one and part of another with a shoulder injury, but he still was named AFC Defensive Rookie of the Year. The following season he started all 16 contests, finishing third on the team with 105 tackles. The Cleveland secondary seemed to be set and probably would even get better as twenty-three-year-old Rogers gained more experience.

In 1986, Hanford Dixon went to California to be part of Rogers' June 28 wedding. The wedding entourage and over twenty other people had a bachelor party for Rogers at the Sacramento Hilton and then went to a local nightclub to continue the celebration until about two in the morning. Afterwards, Rogers went back to the house he had purchased for his mother in an area far from the poor neighborhood he grew up in. Early the next morning, Rogers, after crying out that he was in pain, collapsed into a coma. He never recovered and died at 4:31 pm from cardiac arrest.

An autopsy after Rogers' death showed he had 5.2 milligrams per liter of cocaine in his blood and twice that level in the fluids in his brain. The Sacramento coroner indicated that Rogers had ingested enough cocaine to kill an elephant. The Cleveland defensive star's death came a little more than a week after the Boston Celtic's draftee Len Bias had died of cocaine intoxication.

Several explanations surrounded Rogers' death. One was that he was having a last party before checking into rehab, another was that he was having second thoughts about his marriage, and a third was he was overwhelmed by family matters, including coping with his mother's recent heart attack, with his father's imprisonment for drunk driving, and with supporting a four-year-old son who was the product of a college relationship. No matter how the story was told, the ending was tragic—Rogers was gone and the echoes of his big hits wouldn't be heard in Cleveland again.

PATIENT HISTORY

"He's a vicious tackler, a fearless hitter. He'll really put the leather to you if you're not careful."
—Terry Donahue, UCLA coach

"We can only hope and pray that Don's death makes more people realize the necessity of avoiding drugs,"
—Marty Schottenheimer, Cleveland head coach

"I was supposed to be a groomsman in his wedding on Saturday. Now I will be a pallbearer at his funeral Thursday."
—Kenny Easley

DIAGNOSIS

Don Rogers should have been the centerpiece of the Cleveland Browns defense in the late 1980s. Perhaps he was the missing piece that would have pushed the team from the AFC Championship game to the Super Bowl in 1988 and 1989. During his two years in Cleveland, Rogers was the type of intimidating safety that caused receivers to develop "alligator arms" and drop passes. Opposing receivers learned to stay out of "Mr. Rogers' neighborhood." Browns fans were emotionally distraught by the loss of Rogers, a young and talented defender.

SECOND OPINION

In 1986, without Rogers, the Browns' defense was ranked eleventh in points allowed, after finishing seventh and sixth the previous two seasons respectively. On "The Drive" that ended the Browns' Super Bowl hopes, Rogers might have provided a key play to stop John Elway and the Broncos. The following year, however, the Browns were ranked second in points allowed, but "The Fumble" stopped the team from going to Pasadena for Super Bowl XXI. Still, seeing Rogers matched up against Elway would have been worth the price of admission.

TREATMENT

Cocaine is a powerful central nervous system stimulant with significant cardiovascular side effects, which typically occur within seconds or minutes. Cocaine gives a user a feeling of euphoria. The ancient Incas believed cocaine to be a gift from the gods. Cocaine usage is the third most common cause of drug-related visits to the emergency room in the United States, ranking below only alcohol and tobacco. Other drugs are often present in patients with cocaine toxicity. Signs of intoxication include enlarged pupils, agitation, increased heart rate, and increased blood pressure. Higher doses can produce sweating, tremors, confusion, hyperactivity, seizures, stroke, and cardiac arrhythmias. Many of its dangerous side effects on the heart include reducing blood flow in the coronary arteries, depressing the function of the heart muscle, and causing heart arrhythmias, including arrhythmias (abnormal electrical activity) that produce sudden death.

Effective treatment of cocaine addiction must take into account neurobiological, social, and medical aspects of the patient's drug abuse. Since no FDA-approved medication treats cocaine addiction, the strategies for recovery involve behavioral therapy, residential programs, and community-based recovery groups—such as Cocaine Anonymous. Various sources report relapse rates of over 50 percent after intervention.

INCIDENTAL FINDINGS

A few years after Rogers' death, Kevin Mack, a Browns running back, was arrested for cocaine possession when eleven fifty-dollar bags of crack cocaine were found in his car. He was suspended thirty days by the NFL for violating the NFL's drug policy. Mack eventually pled guilty to only one count of drug abuse and in October 1989 was sentenced to six months in jail. He did return to the Browns and had three productive seasons before retiring.

During the time Rogers played for the Browns, the team had formed a group, the Inner Circle, to help players with drug abuse problems. Started by Coach Sam Rutigliano in 1981, the group was instrumental in helping Charles White recover from his cocaine addiction. Calvin Hill and Paul Warfield were the key contacts for players seeking advice and treatment.

Cashing in the Chip

Michael Wayne "A Mad Dog in a Meat Market" Junkin

Born: 1964
Cleveland Browns: 1987–88
Position: Linebacker
Jersey Number: 54

SYMPTOMS

In 1986, the Cleveland Browns were minutes away from making their first Super Bowl appearance. Denver's John Elway engineered "The Drive" and the Browns lost their bid in overtime. The fans' heartbreak was palpable. Knowing the team could make another run at postseason glory, the Browns turned to the 1987 draft make some improvements.

Mike Junkin, a Duke linebacker, set school records in 1986 for most tackles in a season (188), which garnered him All-ACC and All-American honors. Standing six foot three and weighing 230 pounds, Junkin had suffered a back injury as a sophomore and a knee injury during his junior season, leading some NFL executives to question his durability. However, he ran an impressive time in the forty-yard dash at the draft combine, improving his draft status. Several teams ahead of the Browns, who originally had the twenty-fourth selection, had interest in Junkin, including Oakland, Houston, Minnesota, and Dallas, though most experts still considered the Duke player the fourth or fifth best linebacker prospect.

Sold on the skills of Junkin, the Browns traded All-Pro linebacker Chip Banks and their first two draft picks to the San Diego Chargers for their first two picks to move ahead of the teams interested in Junkin. The Browns were less than enamored with Banks' yearly holdouts, and one official thought that it was time he moved on. With the fifth pick, the Browns chose the "mad dog in the meat market" to play outside linebacker, even though he had always played inside linebacker at Duke. Junkin held out—like Banks might have—and reported to camp late in August, missing much of preseason training.

In 1987, Junkin appeared in only four games, none as a starter, and his season was ended in November by a possible career-threatening wrist injury. Junkin needed six and a half hours of surgery to fix the torn ligaments and dislocation. He had to have several ligaments sewn back together and pins placed in his wrist to aid in healing. Junkin started seven games in 1988, but suffered a sprained knee ligament during the season, forcing him to miss several games. Junkin's career with Cleveland ended in 1989, when he was traded to Kansas City for a fifth-round draft pick. Junkin was out of football after one season with the Chiefs. Rumors later surfaced that the Browns knew that Junkin took steroids during his Duke career, but sources also reported that the use was to aid in the healing process for his ankle injury and not for strengthening purposes.

Junkin's draft has to be considered questionable at best and disastrous at worst. The overall 1987 draft class was not as strong as previous years either, especially at linebacker. The Browns might have been better off drafting Cornelius Bennett, who had a fourteen-year career, Shane Conlan from Penn State, or Winston Moss from Miami.

PATIENT HISTORY

"We had him [Junkin] ranked in the top three players in the country. He is one of the finest college linebackers I have ever seen."
—Marty Schottenheimer, Cleveland head coach

"He's wanted to go back inside in the worst way and they've said, 'No, you're an outside linebacker.' He's been pouting about it ever since."
—Browns source

> "Dubbed 'a mad dog in a meat market,' he [Junkin] was more like a scared French poodle amongst ravenous mountain lions."
> —Steve King, columnist

DIAGNOSIS

The choice of Mike Junkin in the 1987 NFL Draft was highly damaging to the franchise in several ways. The Browns were talented, having gone to the playoffs in the previous two years. The 1986 Cleveland Pro Bowlers included Chip Banks, Bob Golic, Kevin Mack, Clay Matthews, and Ozzie Newsome. In 1987, Chip Banks, Hanford Dixon, Bob Golic, Frank Minnifield, and Cody Risien were chosen as Pro Bowlers. The Browns were a small step away from a Super Bowl appearance and needed only one or two quality players to get the team over the top. Junkin was supposed to help the team get to the opposing quarterback, a deficiency that some considered contributed to the losses to the Denver Broncos.

By trading star linebacker Chip Banks, the Browns created a gaping hole in the defense. Even worse, by selecting Junkin, the Browns passed on a plethora of talent, including defensive tackle Jerome Brown (two-time Pro Bowler), linebacker Shane Conlan (three-time Pro Bowler), and NFL Hall of Fame defensive back Rod Woodson. Clearly the Browns' brass missed out on a "Super" opportunity.

SECOND OPINION

The loss of Banks seemed to be a blow to the defense, but numbers tell a different story; the Browns became better defensively. During the last Banks season (1986–87), the Browns were eleventh in the league in points allowed, giving up 310 points. They sacked the opposing quarterback 35 times. In 1987–88, although the sack total went down by one sack, the team was second in the league in points allowed, giving up only 239 points. The team gave up 288 points the following year and recorded 36 sacks.

Perhaps drafting Junkin was a nearsighted pick since the Browns needed a young quarterback to backup Kosar; Steve Beuerlein, Rich Gannon, and Jim Harbaugh were all available. By the 1988–89 season, Cleveland's offense had fallen to twentieth in the league, scoring only 304 points (they had scored 391 and 390 points the previous two years). While the Browns' front office was convinced Junkin was the answer, maybe the question wasn't framed properly.

TREATMENT

Many injuries to the wrist can be debilitating and career-threatening for athletes. One of the most common sports injuries to the wrist is a fracture to one of the small bones known as the navicular or scaphoid (see medical illustration, page 305). The scaphoid is located on the thumb side of the wrist, near where the wrist bends.

The bone can be easily located with the thumb in the hitchhiker position. The hollow area below the thumb tendon is called the snuffbox; the scaphoid is a C-shaped or canoe-shaped bone directly beneath the snuffbox. The most common cause of the injury is a fall on an outstretched hand. The injury initially presents with swelling and decreased range of motion. After a few days or weeks of improvement, athletes may tape the injury and consider it a sprain.

Unfortunately, there are two major problems with diagnosing scaphoid fractures. First, the fracture often does not show on an X-ray until weeks later. A follow-up X-ray or MRI may be required for a correct diagnosis. Second, if a fracture is undiagnosed, the bone can become a nonunion fracture and never heal properly. Among the causes of nonunion are: infection, insufficient fracture immobilization, and inadequate blood supply, which can lead to avascular necrosis (AVN) or the death of the bone. In nonunion instances, fusion surgery is necessary. After surgery, athletes cannot bend their wrists normally, a condition that can be career-ending, depending on the sport.

Typically a wrist injury, when diagnosed early, can be treated with a cast. However, in certain locations of the bone (areas of the poorest blood flow), the bone is fixed by use of a surgical screw. A newer surgical treatment uses a graft that has its own bloody supply (vascularized graft) and has greatly improved outcomes for athletes.

INCIDENTAL FINDINGS

Medicine has come a long way in dealing with many injuries and ailments. However, it seems that some parts of the body don't heal as well as others; the wrist area seems to be one of them.

> H. S. F., aged twenty, injured his wrist in playing football at Cambridge. He was seen by the surgeon of the football squad and the wrist was put in splints for several days. The swelling and tenderness subsided to a certain extent.... In football practice it is found that a sprain does better if the use of the limb is kept up, and this wrist was treated on this principle. While there was some improvement, the joint still remained sore, forced motions beyond a slight angle were very painful and the gain in strength was slow. About six weeks after the original injury the patient consulted me at my office. I made a diagnosis of fracture of the scaphoid and confirmed it by an X-ray. Feeling that it was too late to endeavor to obtain union between the fractured ends of the bone, I only kept the wrist on splints for about two weeks and then had it massaged. The rest on the splints improved the joint to a considerable extent but it still remained somewhat swollen and gave pain if extreme motions were forced. The young man was prevented from doing any sort of athletics with the wrist; he could not play football, and frequently found that he hurt it in scrapping with the other fellows. This condition has lasted over two years with a very gradual gain, so that even now the wrist cannot be extended beyond an angle of 25° without giving extreme pain. (*Boston Medical and Surgical Journal* 150, no. 14, 1904)

Flagged for Roughing

Orlando Claude "Big Hoss" "Zeus" Brown

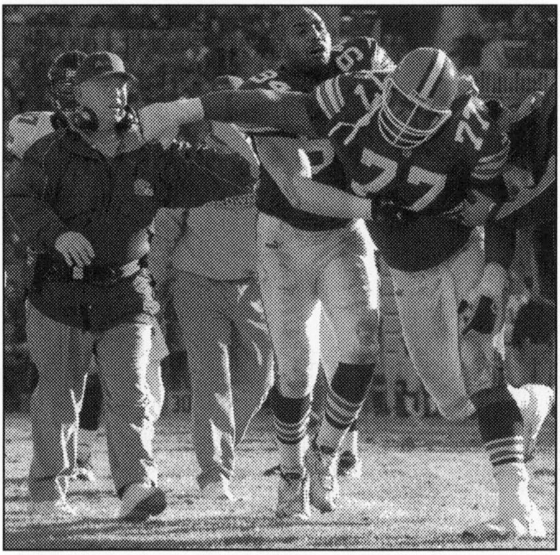

Born: 1970 Died: 2011
Cleveland Browns: 1994–95; 1999
Position: Offensive Tackle
Jersey Number: 77

Orlando Brown tries to get to Jeff Triplette after being hit in the eye with a penalty flag, 1999 (Courtesy *Akron Beacon Journal*)

SYMPTOMS

Though decades apart, Marion Motley, a member of the Pro Football Hall of Fame, and Orlando Brown had some common ties. Both were large men for their eras. Motley, playing in the late 1940s and 1950s, stood six foot one and weighed 232 pounds. Brown weighed around 360 pounds and stood six foot seven during his playing days in the late 1990s. Both men went to South Carolina State University, a predominately black college in Orangeburg, South Carolina, and both were members of the Cleveland Browns.

Orlando Brown grew up on the streets of Washington DC, where drug, guns, and gangs were prevalent. During the funeral of one of Brown's cousins, who had been gunned down in a drive-by shooting, the rival gang shot holes in the coffin, not content with just killing the victim. The constant threat of violence gave Brown a temper that put him over the edge at times.

Orlando Brown was signed as a free agent by the Browns in 1993 after his college career was completed. Nicknamed "Big Hoss" by his teammates, Brown went on to become one of the higher-paid offensive linemen in the NFL. After a 1992 season where Cleveland averaged only 3.6 yards rushing per carry, an improved offensive line was a top priority of Coach Bill Belichick. Brown started his first game in the 1994 season and the Browns completed an 11–5 campaign, winning a Wild-Card Game against New England, but losing in the divisional playoff to Pittsburgh. After starting the 1995 season at 4–4, the Browns lost seven of their last eight games. The downward spiral was completed when Art Modell moved the team to Baltimore.

Brown, starting 69 of 71 regular season games, played with the Ravens until 1999, when the Browns franchise was resurrected in Cleveland. He was re-signed by the team to a six-year, $26-million contract. Late in the 1999 season, Browns fans witnessed a bizarre incident in a December 19 game against the Jacksonville Jaguars that ended Zeus's season and his career with the Browns.

During the second quarter of the game, the referee Jeff Triplette threw a flag to indicate that center Jim Bundrun had moved too early. Unfortunately, the flag—weighted with BBs—went through Brown's faceguard and struck him in the left eye. The big lineman was stunned and taken to the bench, where his eye began to swell shut. Although Triplett apologized, Zeus rushed back onto the field and shoved the referee to the ground. Four security guards led the tackle to the locker room after his automatic ejection.

Many of Brown's teammates were disappointed in his actions, but also were cognizant of the unusual situation that caused the injury. The NFL was less than sympathetic, suspending Brown indefinitely. Cleveland released Brown midseason the following year, after determining that he was not close to being physically able to play.

Brown won a settlement from the NFL in 2001, in the amount of approximately $15–$25 million, contending the Triplette incident ended his career prematurely. The lineman came out of retirement in 2003 and played three seasons with the Ravens. On September

23, 2011, Brown was found dead in his Baltimore apartment of diabetic ketoacidosis—severe complications associated with diabetes.

PATIENT HISTORY

> "I'm ready to play ball. I'm ready to bust some heads and I'm ready to get some W's."
> —Orlando Brown

> "There was no better friend, no one more loyal than Zeus was to his teammates."
> —Ozzie Newsome

> "There is no way to quantify his heart, his actual love to play football."
> —Brian Billick, Ravens coach

DIAGNOSIS

The terribly weak offensive line of the early 1990s was painful to watch for Cleveland fans. The team couldn't run the ball, couldn't stop the run, and couldn't protect Bernie Kosar. Signing Orlando Brown was a good move for Cleveland, intended to fix one of those problems. Brown started 24 games for the team during the 1994 and 1995 seasons. He then followed the team when it moved to Baltimore. The Browns re-signed Zeus when the franchise was resurrected in 1999. Brown, a player who was reaching his peak, was to be a stable fixture on a team of rookies, free agents, and veterans nearing retirement.

What happened to Brown was freakish, improbable, and devastating. The odds of being partially blinded from a penalty flag were unfathomable. Brown's reaction and ejection were bad enough, but the implications to his health made the incident tragic. Financially, Brown's injury had unfortunate implications; not only did it affect the team's salary cap, but it limited the ability to sign higher-priced free agents. Even after the team cut Brown, the financial repercussions lingered for several years.

The bizarre incident in the Browns' return to the lakefront didn't bode well. Was the incident an indicator of a "haunted" franchise? Were the gods of football making a statement regarding the team's chances of improving quickly and regaining past glory? Fans seemed to be muttering "Why us? Why now?"

SECOND OPINION

Even if Orlando "Zeus" Brown had returned and played in 2000, the offensive line would not have been much better. The 1999 linemen didn't seem to have the ability to compete at the NFL level. An aging Lomas Brown went to the New York Giants, Scott Rehberg went to Cincinnati, and Chris Ruhman was out of football after the 1999 season. Jim Pyne (see page 173), Steve Zahursky, and Jim Bundren lasted one more year and were never heard from again. Orlando Bobo became a backup for Baltimore for two years. Only Dave Wohlabaugh and Roger Chanoine played with the team through the 2002 season. The team's brass wasn't very good at picking talent through the draft, either. Even when game-time weather was nice, dark clouds were draped over the team's development.

TREATMENT

An injury that causes bleeding in the anterior chamber of the eye is known as a hyphema (see medical illustration, page 297). The blood generally settles to the lower part of the eye, creating "fluid level" or straight top, which is clearly visible when looking at the eye. In cases of small hyphemas, eye specialists may only be able to detect the injury with special tool.

Treating the injury quickly results in

- hastening the absorption of blood from the anterior chamber;

- preventing recurrent bleeding;
- preventing or controlling such complications as glaucoma, corneal blood staining, and iritis; and
- treating associated ocular injuries, if present.

Usually the treatment requires complete bed rest, often with hospitalization, in hopes that the injury will resolve on its own. About 15–20 percent of people with a hyphema have further bleeding in the first week after the injury. In some cases, surgery is required. Without treatment, patients will not only suffer pain, but the hyphema might lead to acute glaucoma and impaired vision.

INCIDENTAL FINDINGS

When referees officiated football games in the early years of the sport, a horn was blown when a player violated the rules. Eventually, whistles replaced horns to indicate infractions, but players began to confuse whistles to stop play with whistles that indicated penalties. In 1941, the penalty flag was born at a game between Youngstown University and Oklahoma City University.

Dwight Beede, the coach of the Youngstown team, had his wife Irma sew together red and white flags for the contest. With the cooperation of the OCU coach and the officials, the flags were thrown onto the field when an infraction occurred. One of the officials used the flags at another game and the practice caught on. The flags were eventually changed to yellow to make them more distinguishable. Beede would end up seeing many officials toss penalty flags onto college football fields; he coached the YSU Penguins from 1938–74.

Booed and Belittled

Timothy Scott "Ouch" Couch

Born: 1977
Cleveland Browns:
1999–2003
Position: Quarterback
Jersey Number: 2

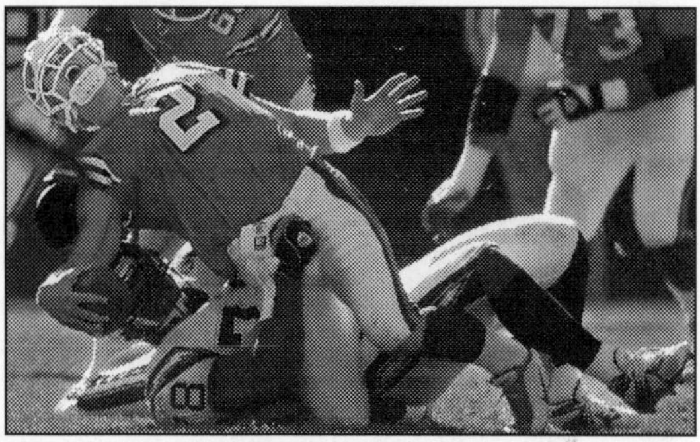

Tim Couch takes a painful sack versus San Diego, 2003 (Courtesy *Akron Beacon Journal*)

SYMPTOMS

Tim Couch was a two-sport phenom during his high school years at Leslie County in rural Kentucky. The eighteen-year-old, standing six foot five and weighing 215 pounds, led the state in scoring on the basketball court during his junior year, averaging 36 points a game. However, he was even more sought after by college football recruiters because he reminded them of John Elway. Couch, who grew up in Hyden, was so impressive on the gridiron that fans came from all over Kentucky to watch him play.

Couch went on to the University of Kentucky and led his team to the Outback Bowl in his junior season. Couch still holds the record for most completions in a season, most yards passing in a season, and best completion percentage at Kentucky. He was a Heisman finalist in his junior year, losing out to Ricky Williams of Texas. Instead of staying at UK, he declared himself eligible for the 1999 draft and the Browns, returning to the league after a three-year hiatus, chose the Kentucky star with the first overall pick.

The unfortunate combination of fan expectations and the reality of being on an expansion team plagued Couch over his career, which lasted until 2003. Couch, to put it mildly, was never admired by the Cleveland fans. Perhaps impatience had built up over the years when Clevelanders couldn't go to the lakefront to watch games. The 1999 Browns finished with a 2–14 record, the 2000 team won three games, and although the Browns went 7–9 in 2001, Couch still faced criticism.

To his credit, Couch led the team to the 2002 playoffs after sitting out several early season games with an elbow injury and as later reported, fraying in his rotator cuff. On his return against the Baltimore Ravens, trailing 23–8 in the fourth quarter, Couch was knocked in the back of the head and suffered a concussion. As he lay on the field fans began to cheer, realizing Kelly Holcomb would replace Couch. After that contest, which the Browns lost 26–21, Couch tearfully ripped into the Cleveland fans. Although many local sportswriters noted that the Browns' defense was flawed and the team had no running game to speak of, Browns Coach Butch Davis didn't provide full support for the embattled quarterback.

Couch came back the next week against Tampa Bay and over the last eleven games of the season the team went 7–4. In the regular season finale against the Atlanta Falcons, Couch suffered a broken leg. His backup, Kelly Holcomb, started against the Steelers in the playoffs and even though the Browns suffered a bitter defeat, Holcomb completed 26 of 43 passes for 429 yards and 3 touchdowns.

Kelly Holcomb became the Browns starter in 2003. The Browns made no secret of the fact that Couch was available, but questions about his broken leg, arm strength, and his salary dissuaded teams from making any offers to the Browns. In the end, due to an injury Holcomb suffered in 2003, both quarterbacks started eight games and the team finished at 5–11. Before the 2004 season, Tim Couch was released by the Browns because they had signed thirty-four-year-old Jeff Garcia to be their quarterback. The Browns' first overall draft pick was now last in the minds of Cleveland fans.

PATIENT HISTORY

"We just didn't have a lot of talent. Every week was a struggle. Then I had my problems. I kept getting hurt. It was one thing after another."
—Tim Couch

"Somewhere along the line, Tim Couch has to play. Whether it's today, tomorrow, next year, he has to play. But he'll also go through a growing process when he steps on the field."
—Chris Palmer, Browns coach during Couch's rookie season

"Either you're going to be with us or you're going to be against us, and you're not helping us at all if you're sitting there booing one [Couch] of these players on this team"
—Daylon McCutcheon, Browns cornerback

DIAGNOSIS

Fans were overflowing with anticipation prior to the 1999 NFL Draft because the Browns had the number one overall pick. There was no doubt that the team would come away with a great player, but fans expected the team to select a great quarterback, maybe a future Hall of Famer. Tim Couch was chosen as the cornerstone of the team and was considered the prototypical big quarterback with a strong arm who would lead the Browns to the Super Bowl. He was destined to make big plays and revive a storied franchise.

After an opening day 43–0 massacre by the Pittsburgh Steelers, the Browns thrust their $48-million, touchdown-throwing machine into the fray. Unfortunately, Couch was sacked 56 times and the team scored 217 points during the season, last in the league. The rushing game was abysmal, too.

Looking back, Couch was forced into a terrible situation early in his career; he wasn't ready and neither were any of the offensive pieces around him. The fans will always wonder whether Couch had first overall pick skills or if the state of the team ruined his confidence and his body. The culmination of the team's roller-coaster ride was the night he suffered a concussion during a nationally televised 2002 game against the Baltimore Ravens. Couch was so emotional in the postgame interview that he broke down and cried; the courtship, honeymoon, and marriage between the Browns and Tim Couch ended after that game.

SECOND OPINION

The Browns weren't alone in picking a quarterback in the first round of the 1999 draft. Donovan McNabb went at number two to the Eagles, Akili Smith (Bengals) was the third overall pick, Daunte Culpepper went to the Vikings with the eleventh overall selection, and Chicago chose Cade McNown twelfth. While it wouldn't have been popular, the team would have been better off drafting offensive or defensive linemen with their picks.

The following year, the Browns chose Courtney Brown with the number one overall pick and he also turned out to be a bust. The rest of the 2000 draft class didn't pan out in any substantial way. In 2001, with the third overall pick, the team chose Gerard Warren. His addition, along with other picks that year, didn't provide much quality. Talent evaluation, obviously, didn't yield any talent.

TREATMENT

In Couch's case, the likely injury was a frontal lobe concussion. The brain's frontal lobe controls emotions, and if damaged, an individual is not able to control feelings or impulses. In some instances, repeated minor frontal lobe injuries can cause damage to the brain's "executive function," which includes organizational functions like planning, sequencing, problem solving, and abstract thinking, and regulatory functions like self-control, emotional regulation, moral reasoning, and decision making. Also, see Mark Price, page 244; Colt McCoy, page 201; and medical illustration, page 295.

INCIDENTAL FINDINGS

Recently, concussions and their long-lasting effects have taken center stage. However, the dangers of concussions were evident early in the twentieth century. Equipment was not as advanced in the pioneering days of football, but players were also not as physically gifted.

> This portion of the report [*The Physical Aspect of American Football*] is so important as a reflection on the results that may follow from a sport that we quote it as it is given:
>
> Cases of concussion were frequent, both during practice and games. In fact, but two games were played during the entire season in which a case of concussion of the brain did not occur. There were several noticeable features in these cases. Frequently, the fact that a man has received a serious head injury was noticed by the surgeon from the side lines before it was recognized by the players. This was due to the fact that a player might, apparently, automatically run thru a considerable series of plays before his mates noticed that he was mentally irresponsible. The mental state of the players who had concussion was variable, some being highly excitable and hysterical, others merely confused, and in a few cases, knocked completely unconscious. In every case there was a certain loss of memory, both previous and subsequent to the injury. . . .
>
> It is no wonder, then, that in their [Dr. Edward H. Nichols and Dr. Homer B. Smith] conclusion the Harvard surgeons should announce that the number, severity and permanency of the injuries received in football are very much greater than generally is credited or believed; that the number of injuries is inherent to the game itself, is not due to close competition, since the proportion is about the same in games and in practice; that a large percentage of the injuries is unavoidable and incomparably greater in football than in any other of the major sports, and that finally the percentage of injury is much too great for any mere sport. (*The Independent*, 1906)

A Buckeye for a Heart

Charles Christopher "Chris" Spielman

Born: 1965
Cleveland Browns: Never played in a regular season game
Position: Linebacker
Jersey Number: 54

SYMPTOMS

Chris Spielman epitomizes the Ohio football hero. Born in Canton, the home of the Pro Football Hall of Fame, Spielman played for the Massillon Tigers, the team once coached by the legendary Paul Brown. Spielman was a *Parade* All-American and as a high schooler gained the national spotlight by being featured on the front of a Wheaties cereal box. Spielman went on to play at Ohio State, where he became an All-American and winner of the 1987 Lombardi Award as the best linebacker in college football.

The Detroit Lions drafted Spielman in the second round (the twenty-ninth pick overall) because there were some worries that he might be too small to play in the NFL. He proved doubters wrong by being named to the Pro Bowl in 1990, 1991, 1992, and 1995. After eight years in Detroit, Spielman was signed to a four-year free agent contract by the Buffalo Bills and made an immediate impact by setting a team record of 206 tackles in 1996. The next season ended in late October for Spielman after he sustained a neck injury and required neck fusion surgery. After taking the 1998 season off to aid in the recovery of his wife, who underwent breast cancer surgery, the Browns traded a low draft choice to Buffalo and signed Spielman to a three-year contract. He was to be part of the 1999 Browns, the rebirth of the franchise that Art Modell had moved to Baltimore several years earlier.

At thirty-four years old, Spielman wasn't going to provide a long-term solution for the team, but his experience and character would be invaluable in the locker room. Spielman had also assured the team that he would know when to hang up his cleats, so management wouldn't have to face fan ire if his skills deteriorated greatly. Unfortunately, the storybook ending never came for Spielman. In an exhibition game against the Chicago Bears, he took a blindside hit while defending a screen pass and lay partially paralyzed on the turf for about fifteen seconds. Eventually, he was able to walk off the field and out of the stadium for the last time.

PATIENT HISTORY

> "For me as a northeast Ohio kid to play my last game on the Cleveland Browns field, in front of Cleveland Browns fans, in a Cleveland Browns helmet. You couldn't write it any better,"
> —Chris Spielman

> "[Spielman] was straight throwback; Dick Butkus, Ray Nitschke—that was this guy. He was cut out of that mold."
> —Lomas Brown, Detroit Lion teammate

> "Chris Spielman is the most intense player I have ever seen. He has the rare quality of being able to make a great play in a critical situation."
> —Earle Bruce, Ohio State head coach

DIAGNOSIS

Chris Spielman was the ideal football player to lead the new Browns defense in 1999. His legendary toughness and ferocious style of play typified the region, the city, and the glory days of the team. Before the season started, many Browns fans hurried to purchase Spielman jerseys. His comeback wasn't ever to be realized, however, as Spielman brought injury baggage from many years of football, which included hundreds of tackles. He collided with Chicago Bears center Casey Wiegmann and reinjured his neck during a preseason game. Despite the seriousness of his injury, he refused to be carried off, typifying his demeanor on the field. After having already gone through a serious spinal fusion surgery, Spielman was forced to retire, never having played a single down in a regular season game for the Cleveland Browns.

Spielman returned home to his wife Stephanie and his four children. He stood by his wife for ten years while she battled through four bouts with breast cancer. Ultimately, Stephanie lost her battle on November 19, 2009, after her cancer returned for a fifth time. After her death, The Ohio State University renamed their breast cancer facility the Stefanie Spielman Comprehensive Breast Center in honor of the family's contribution to breast cancer research. The Spielman family became great advocates for the cause and they inspired thousands of people to help find a cure.

SECOND OPINION

The Browns selected Rahim Abdullah, an outside linebacker from Clemson, with their third pick in the 1999 draft. Abdullah had been the 1997 Peach Bowl MVP and was selected as an All-Atlantic Coast Conference player in 1998. Abdullah's character wasn't spotless, however, he had been arrested on gun charges and had a few other minor problems. Still, the Browns signed him to a five-year, $3-million contract with a $940,000 signing bonus.

Banking on the further development of Abdullah after his rookie season, the Browns did not select a linebacker in the 2000 draft. Among the available linebackers were Brian Urlacher, LaVar Arrington, Julian Peterson, and Na'il Diggs from Ohio State University. Abdullah had a few injuries in the 2000 season, never developed, and was off the squad before the next training camp.

TREATMENT

According to various studies, between 600,000 and 1.2 million football-related injuries occur annually in the United States. Ten to twenty-five percent of the injuries involve the spine or axial skeleton (the bones forming the axis of the skeleton, including the skull, vertebrae, ribs, and sternum). The National Football League has recently taken action to improve player safety by penalizing hits on defenseless players and imposing restrictions on using the helmet in spearing.

The stinger or burner, a cervical spine injury, occurs in 20 percent to 25 percent of professional football players in a given season. Known by the medical term brachio plexopathy, the injury occurs from a significant stretching or bruising to the nerves in the neck, causing a burning sensation in the arm. An athlete usually complains of pain that radiates from the neck to the hand. They also complain of weakness, and often after injury, their arms dangle at their sides. Usually, the injury lasts for a short period of time. However, in cases when the injury recurs or is more serious, the condition can last for months and might cause permanent damage.

A more severe football injury is called spinal stenosis—the narrowing of the spinal canal where the spinal cord resides. Stenosis can be caused by recurrent injury to bones, including fractures, by arthritis or by recurrent disc injuries. Spinal stenosis might put football players at a greater risk for paralyzing neck injuries.

A long list of congenital abnormalities to the spine can preclude athletes from competing in a hard-hitting sport like football, because of the risk of permanent paralyzing injuries.

Because of the nature of spinal injuries, an athlete's return to play must be considered with care. The following list indicates three levels of management scenarios that can be used to determine whether an athlete should resume competition.

- No contraindications (to give indication against the advisability of a certain action) or full return to play. This category includes players who have had stingers, but who have recovered completely.

- Relative contraindications for return to play. The second group includes players with chronic recurrent stingers with incomplete neurologic recovery. Athletes who have fully healed (having no persistent nerve symptoms) after spine fusion surgery or single-level disc surgery fall into this category. In this scenario, the athlete must understand the risk of reinjury is uncertain.
- Absolute contraindications to return to play. Athletes with decreased range of motion from the condition known as Spear Tackler's Spine (see Incidental Findings below) or from certain congenital abnormalities are included in this category. Returning to play is dissuaded.

INCIDENTAL FINDINGS

Spear Tackler's Spine (STS) was originally described in 1993 in athletes who frequently tackled opponents using their head gear. These athletes exhibited the following characteristics:

- developmental narrowing of the cervical spinal canal;
- straightening or reversal of the normal inward curvature of the lumbar and cervical regions of the spine curve; and
- preexisting posttraumatic X-ray evidence of bone or ligament injury.

Most caregivers insist that athletes who exhibit spear tackler's spine should not return to contact or collision sports (*American Journal of Sports Medicine* 21, no. 5 (1993): 640–49).

Spearing gained infamy during a 1970 game between bitter rivals Kansas City and Oakland. Late in the contest, Ben Davidson of Oakland dove headfirst onto Kansas City's quarterback Len Dawson as he lay facedown on the ground after a first down. Dawson took the blow in the small of the back. Bob Dates of the *Los Angeles Times* described the incident as using the helmet or head as a weapon to "spear" a defenseless player on the ground.

His Achilles Heel

Jamir Malik Miller

Born: 1973
Cleveland Browns: 1999–2001
Position: Linebacker
Jersey Number: 95

SYMPTOMS

Jamir Miller always wanted to get better. His mother tells a story of him sounding out words in the newspaper at three so he could understand what was going on. Miller was born in Baltimore, but his father was a drug addict and his mother moved the family to Oakland, California. Miller couldn't avoid all the gang-related activities, but his mother forced him out of the area by making him attend the safer, suburban El Cerrito High School. The move was instrumental in getting him on the football field, where he excelled.

Miller, a top high school linebacker, also ran track. He went on to star at UCLA, though he did have several off-field incidents that tarnished his reputation. His athletic talent was never in doubt and Miller was chosen tenth overall by the Arizona Cardinals in the 1994 NFL Draft. While with Arizona, Miller played in every game between 1994 and 1998, with the exception of a six-game stretch in 1995 due to a league-implemented four-game suspension after violating the substance abuse policy.

One spectacular play highlighted Miller's time with Arizona. In a game against the Detroit, Barry Sanders of the Lions, a 2004 Hall of Fame inductee, burst into the open and headed for what looked like a sure touchdown. Miller, however, outsprinted him and tackled him. At six foot five and weighing 266 pounds, Miller was deceptively fast.

Instead of accepting a new contract with the Cardinals, the twenty-six-year-old Miller signed with Cleveland midseason in 1999. He became an impactful player, leading the team with 117 tackles and adding 4.5 sacks. He started 47 of his 48 games with Cleveland and was named to the 2001 Pro Bowl after recording 83 solo tackles and 13 sacks.

When the Browns gathered for training camp for the 2002 season, a renewed optimism seemed to surround the defense. Even if Miller didn't match his 2001 statistics, he was still going to be a force other teams would have to plan around. After an August 10 preseason game against the Minnesota Vikings, Miller came out of the locker room on crutches and was taken to the team bus in a golf cart. He had ruptured his right Achilles tendon in the first quarter, which ended up being his last quarter with the Browns and in the NFL. After sitting out the entire 2002 season and still experiencing pain in his injured foot, Miller retired from the game in May 2003. The void left at outside linebacker contributed to a 5–11 season and thoughts of how many more times Miller might have made it to the Pro Bowl.

PATIENT HISTORY

"I think he will definitely come in and be a force. He's going to be a playmaker on defense."
—Chris Palmer, Browns coach

"We lost the best outside linebacker in the AFC."
—Dwayne Rudd, Browns linebacker

"His unfortunate Achilles injury kept him off the field during our playoff run last season, but we will always remember the significant contributions he made during our formative years."
—Carmen Policy, Browns president

DIAGNOSIS

Jamir Miller was a phenomenal athlete nearing the top of his game when he suffered his career-ending injury. He had three elite seasons after joining the new Browns in 1999; however, injuries are always an unknown. Even after he sustained a significant Achilles rupture, the Cleveland faithful hoped Jamir Miller would return and chase down opponents again, but his comeback was not in the cards.

SECOND OPINION

In hindsight, the midseason signing of Jamir Miller was not successful. But did the Browns need to be so quick in offering Miller an extended contract? The Browns got Miller at a bargain salary because many teams didn't want to take a chance on the Arizona Cardinal. He had tested positive twice for substance abuse, which meant he was facing a season-long suspension if he strayed one more time.

True, Miller could have tried the free-agent market after the 1999 season, but other teams might have had the same indifference to signing the linebacker. The Browns inked a contract that provided a $6-million signing bonus and a four-year extension worth $18 million. Perhaps the Browns knew Miller was the only true star on a team that had just returned to the league. The amount Miller received, however, might have been better appropriated to free agents who would have been available after the season.

TREATMENT

The Achilles tendon (see medical illustration, page 314) is one of the strongest shock absorbers in the body. Professional athletes, especially those in sports requiring explosive acceleration, sudden changes in direction, or extreme effort, are more prone to Achilles tendon ruptures. When the tendon ruptures, an individual often feels like she/he has been violently kicked or shot in the back of the ankle. Tendon ruptures can occur early in an athletic endeavor if an athlete has not warmed up properly or later in a contest when an athlete is fatigued. The injury to an Achilles tendon suddenly puts athletes in career-threatening predicaments.

While conservative treatments are available, athletes usually face surgery in order for them to return to sports activity. Surgical techniques, including open repair, percutaneous (effected through the skin), and miniopen repair, are available to allow athletes to regain normal function, strength, and range of motion. In general, postoperative rehabilitation can take from nine months to a year.

Unfortunately, upwards of 30 percent of athletes who suffer Achilles ruptures do not return to play. Results of a 2009 article that studied Achilles ruptures in the NFL population indicated that even when a player returned to the field, he was, on average, about 50 percent less effective than prior to surgery. Before injury, the players studied averaged participation in almost twelve games a season. After injury and rehabilitation, they played in only six games a season on average (*Foot Ankle Specialist* 19 (Dec. 2009): 283–86).

INCIDENTAL FINDINGS

Monro's bandage and splint to treat Achilles tendon rupture, circa 1700.

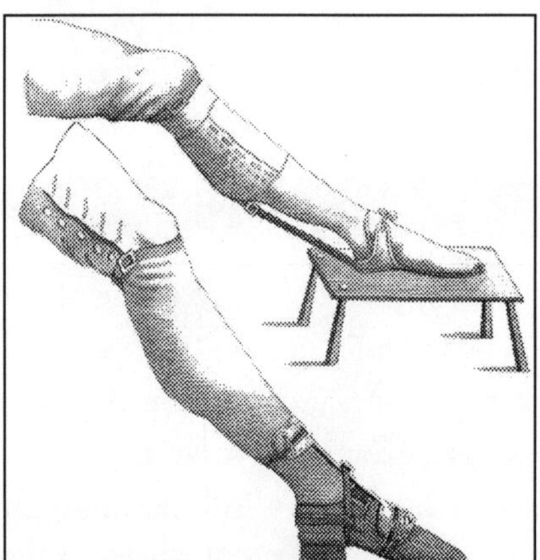

Illustration of Monro's bandage.

The celebrated Dr. Alexander Monro, professor of anatomy at Edinburgh, happened to rupture his tendo Achillis. When the accident took place, he heard a loud crack, as if he had suddenly broken a nut with his heel, and he experienced a sensation, as if the heel of his shoe had made a hole in the floor. This sensation, he says, has also been observed by others, though some have complained of a smart stroke, like what would be produced by a stone or cane. Immediately suspecting what had happened, the doctor extended his left foot, in which the occurrence had taken place, as strongly as he could with his right hand, while with the left, he pressed the muscles of the calf downward, so as to bring the ends of the broken tendon as near together as possible.

> In this position he sat, until two surgeons came to his assistance. They applied compresses, and a bent board to the upper part of the foot, and forepart of the leg, both which they kept, as nearly as possible, in a straight line, by a tight bandage, made with a long roller. But, as this mode of dressing soon became very uneasy, it was changed for the following one. A footsock, or slipper, was made of double quilted ticking, from the heel of which a belt or strap projected, of sufficient length to come up over the calf of the leg. A strong piece, of the same materials, was prepared of sufficient breadth to surround the calf, and this was fastened with lacings. On the back part of this was a buckle, through which the strap of the footsock was passed, so that the foot could be extended, and the calf brought down at pleasure. The leg and foot were wrapt up in soft flannel, fumigated with benzoin, and the bandage was kept on day and night, the belt being made tighter, when the doctor was about to go to sleep, and loosened when he was awake, and on his guard. For a fortnight, he did not move his foot and leg at all, but, was conveyed in a chair on castors from one part of the room to another.
>
> After this, he began to move the ankle joint, but in such a gentle manner as not to give any pain. The degree of motion was gradually increased, as the tendon became capable, of bearing it, care being taken to stop, when the motion began to create

uneasiness. The affected limb was moved in this way for half an hour at a time. In a few days, the hollow, between the separated ends of the tendon, became imperceptible, though the part continued soft much longer. It became, however, gradually thicker and harder until a knot was at last formed in it, apparently of cartilaginous nature. Though this was at first as large as a middling plum, and gradually became softer and smaller yet.

Having occasion to go out six weeks after the accident, the doctor put on a pair of shoes, with heels two inches high, and contrived a steel machine to keep his foot in the proper position. This machine, however, he afterwards changed for another, made of the same materials as the former. It was not till five months after the accident, that he thought proper to lay aside all assistance, and to put the strength of the tendon to trial. (Samuel Cooper, *A Dictionary of Practical Surgery*, 3rd ed., Longman, 1818)

Torn and Tattered

James M. "Jim" Pyne

Born: 1971
Cleveland Browns: 1999–2001
Position: Offensive Guard
Jersey Number: 71

SYMPTOMS

Jim Pyne was born with football in his blood. His grandfather played for the Providence Steam Roller and his father was a defensive tackle for the Boston Patriots. Pyne, after attending Choate Rosemary Hall in Connecticut, became the first unanimous All-American at Virginia Tech, playing center for the Hokies. The Tampa Bay Buccaneers chose the lineman in the seventh round of the 1994 draft. After several years with Tampa Bay, Pyne was signed by the Lions as an unrestricted free agent and started all sixteen games for them in 1998. Unhappy that the Lions' coach Bobby Ross didn't defend the offensive line from criticism, Pyne asked to be put on the expansion list the following year.

The Browns took Pyne as the first pick in the 1999 expansion draft, hoping the veteran would anchor the offensive line for several years. The six-foot-two, 297-pounder played every snap as the Browns went 2–14 in their return to the NFL. Pyne's career with the Browns didn't last long. In 2000, in practice prior to the second regular season game against the Bengals, Pyne sprained his left ankle and had to be helped off the field. Despite the pain, he started against Cincinnati. After a second-quarter touchdown pass from Tim Couch to tight end Mark Campbell, Pyne tore the anterior cruciate ligament in his right knee while celebrating. He said later that he was in so much pain during the game, that he had likely injured the knee on another play, but the knee gave out after the touchdown.

Pyne underwent season-ending knee surgery, came back for the following training camp, but was released by the team before the season. He was signed by Philadelphia and only started one of their first five games before calling it quits.

PATIENT HISTORY

> "I think Jim is going to be a first-class center in the National Football League. He's very strong, he handles the bull rush very well."
> —Bobby Ross, Detroit Lions head coach

> "I was in a lot of pain during the game. The final thing was when I planted, and my knee gave out."
> —Jim Pyne

> "He's very productive and efficient, but his size is a big negative."
> —Pro football scout

DIAGNOSIS

Even though players available to the Browns in the 1999 expansion draft weren't of high caliber, fans were still excited to see a new Browns team being built. (In hindsight, Kurt Warner could have been drafted by the club.) Jim Pyne signaled that the Browns were building from the ground up. Pyne, the first of the "new" Browns, was a down-in-the-trenches "big ugly" whose character matched Cleveland's hardworking, blue-collar ethic. Pyne turned out to be an above-average starter on an offensive line that was vulnerable at almost every other position.

The team was aiming for a much-improved second season, but the foundation began to crumble in week two. In a moment of celebration following a rare touchdown, Pyne tore his ACL and was out for the season. He never started for the Browns again, and the team was forced to perform reconstructive surgery on its offensive line. Losing the number one choice in the expansion draft to a career-ending injury, coupled with Orlando Brown's eye injury, put Cleveland's quarterbacks and running backs at risk.

SECOND OPINION

By the start of the 2004 season, not one player chosen in the expansion draft was a member of the Browns. Jim Pyne was at best an average center. After he left the Detroit Lions, he was replaced by Mike Compton, a left guard who was moved to the center position. With Pyne at center in 1998, the Lions gave up 45 sacks. In other words, the Lions' strength was not the guys in the trenches.

Basically, building a team through the expansion draft was not a real option. NFL franchises did not leave quality players on their unprotected lists. The expectation that the Browns could build a winner right out of the gate was unrealistic. Without any real depth at key positions, the "new" Browns were well behind all the "old" teams of the National Football League.

TREATMENT

A torn anterior cruciate ligament (ACL) (see medical illustration, page 312) strikes fear in all athletes in sports where making use of lateral movements and quick stopping and starting are keys to performance. The most common occurrence of the injury involves an "awkward collapse," or a twist of the knee. More than 70 percent of ACL injuries are noncontact injuries. During this awkward twisting, the ligament becomes trapped in the bony notch of the thighbone or femur. The ligament can then tear by severing or rupturing in the middle, without being pulled off any bony attachments. ACL injuries most often occur with a "plant, twist, pop" mechanism.

Treatment options for ACL injuries vary, but for elite athletes whose sports require quick cutting ability, in most cases, surgery is required. Swimmers and cyclists may be able to recover with only physical therapy and rehabilitation. Once the ACL tears, repairing it is not a suitable option and reconstructive surgery is required. Using arthroscopic techniques, typically a graft from the patellar tendon (the tendon that attaches the bottom of the kneecap to the top of the shinbone) or the hamstring tendon is used to replace the torn ligament. Rehabilitation after surgery commonly takes six months or longer.

INCIDENTAL FINDINGS

ACL treatment is not a new phenomenon. As early as 1853, Amedeé Bonnet, a professor of surgery at Lyon University, had designed an apparatus to treat knee injuries. The morbidity rate for surgery during the latter nineteenth century precluded operations for knee ligament damage. Early in the twentieth century, a surgeon in Germany devised a technique to suture the ligament with aluminum-bronze wire and pull it tight. This type of repair was improved and remained an option into the early 1980s. The first complete graft reconstruction of the ACL was performed by Ernest William Hey Groves at the General Hospital in Bristol, England. Dr. Langworthy of Spokane, Washington, is attributed with using a patellar tendon to graft a torn ACL in the 1920s. By the late 1970s and early 1980s, the use of the patellar tendon to graft the ACL was becoming widespread and continues to be used today. (Oliver S. Schindler, "Surgery for Anterior Cruciate Ligament Deficiency: A Historical Perspective," *Knee Surgery, Sports Traumatology, Arthroscopy* 20, no. 1 (January 2012): 5–47)

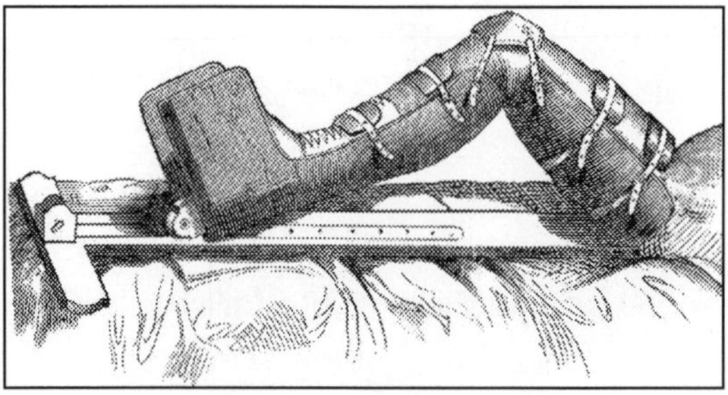

Bonnet's device (1853) enabled movement and prevented stiffness during knee injury rehabilitation

A Storm That Dissipated Quickly

Courtney Lanair "The Quiet Storm" Brown

Born: 1978
Cleveland Browns: 2000–04
Position: Defensive End
Jersey Number: 92

SYMPTOMS

Courtney Brown grew up in a small hamlet, Alvin, in South Carolina. When Brown was selected by Cleveland as the first overall pick in the 2000 draft, Alvin wasn't even on the official state road map and hadn't been since 1956. Brown put together a stellar career at Penn State; the All-American shattered school records for career tackles for loss (70) and sacks (33) and the season mark for tackles for loss (29). He was chosen as the 1999 Big Ten Defensive Player of the Year. Pro scouts compared Brown to Hall of Famer Bruce Smith.

At six foot five and weighing 269 pounds, Brown was projected to be the cornerstone of Cleveland's newly minted defensive line. He received a $10.8-million signing bonus and a six-year, $45-million contract. During his rookie season, Brown started all 16 games and recorded 70 tackles and 4.5 sacks.

The Cleveland organization hoped Brown would show even more dominance during 2001. After a routine training camp, Brown slightly tore the posterior cruciate ligament in his right knee in the last preseason game in late August. He was out for an extensive period of time, returned later in the season, but suffered a high left ankle sprain in a December loss against Tennessee.

In the following years, Brown's injuries continued to pile up—knee and neck injuries in 2002; a torn biceps in 2003; a left foot injury in 2004. Brown underwent surgeries on his right knee in 2001 and his left knee in 2002 and 2004. By December 2002, Brown had missed thirteen games in Butch Davis's two years as the Browns coach. Over his career, which included time with the Denver Broncos, Courtney Brown sat out more games (51) than he played (44).

Brown, who was supposed to bust through offensive lines and sack opposing quarterbacks, was just a plain bust. He had 9 sacks in his first two years with Cleveland and 6 in 2003, but he never started all 16 games after his rookie year. The Browns released him in 2004 for performance and salary-cap reasons.

PATIENT HISTORY

"He's a freak of nature. A guy that big shouldn't be that fast."
—University of Akron football player

"He's an outstanding football player. He's a throwback. . . . When he sacks the quarterback you are not going to see him dance or jaw with someone. He plays the game the way it is meant to be played."
—Chris Palmer, Browns coach

"This is the next Bruce Smith. I'll bet money on it."
—John Wooten, Baltimore Ravens assistant director of pro personnel

DIAGNOSIS

The bad news after the Browns returned to the league in 1999 was that they ended up with the worst record in the league. The good news was that they had the first choice in the 2000 NFL Draft; perhaps a difference maker would be coming to the shores of Lake Erie.

Courtney Brown was a dream athlete; he had a tremendous college career and possessed all the tools to become a dominant professional. One fact about Brown intrigued the draft brain trust of the Cleveland franchise—Brown was injury-free during his college days, playing in every game as a freshman and starting every game from that point on. He was exceptional on the field and in the classroom. Those who knew him and played with him raved about his character. As his frustrating injury story played out, however, the young man known as "The Quiet Storm" simply became silent. The Browns developed a reputation for drafting "sure things" that ended up as "failed selections."

SECOND OPINION

Dwight Clark, the Browns' director of football operations from 1999 through early 2002, is best known for "The Catch" of a Joe Montana pass in the 1981 NFC Championship game. As an NFL executive, he didn't snag much talent for the reincarnated Browns. Of nineteen Browns players who appeared in two or more games in 1999, none played a game in 2000. Of the Browns' twenty-four draft selections in 1999 and 2000, the team drafted only two offensive linemen, one in round six and one in round seven. Browns' President Carmen Policy brought Dwight Clark with him from San Francisco, along with a 49ers-style offense. Unfortunately, Chris Palmer, the coach at the time, came from the Bill Parcells school of football, not the Bill Walsh one.

TREATMENT

Knee injuries are very common in professional sports. Recurrent injuries to the shock-absorbing cartilage pad, known as the meniscus, often occur when planting the foot and turning. Because the majority of the meniscus does not have a blood supply, when it is torn it does not heal on its own and requires surgery to trim, repair, or remove cartilage, depending on the level of damage.

The meniscus is a key protector of the lining surface of the knee joint known as the articular cartilage. For many athletes, recurrent injuries to the meniscus can cause it to wear out prematurely. Prior to the 1990s, this injury would steadily lead to a downhill course toward degenerative arthritis, and in some cases, require total knee replacement. Microfracture surgery, developed in the late 1990s, involves drilling a series of small holes into the articular cartilage (the lining of the joint) to stimulate healing and new cartilage growth.

For professional athletes, the success rate for microfracture surgery (see medical illustration, page 311) varies greatly and this type of surgery is used with great caution. According to the American Orthopaedic Society for Sports Medicine, meniscus surgery can result in a shorter recovery time than ACL surgery. However, players who have had meniscus surgery end up playing fewer games and have significantly shorter careers.

INCIDENTAL FINDINGS

A small enclave on the Santee River Road has no right to produce the 1999 Big Ten Defensive Player of the Year and the 1999 Atlantic Coast Conference Player of the Year. Alvin, South Carolina, can claim that honor. Courtney Brown went to Macedonia High, along with another player, Joe Hamilton, who would go on to star at Georgia Tech. Hamilton threw 99 touchdowns in his high school career, and during his senior year he threw 176 passes without an interception. Hamilton's pro career was as a backup, primarily with Tampa Bay, but he did get a 2002 Super Bowl ring as the team's number three quarterback. After leaving the NFL, Hamilton ended up playing arena football and led his team, the Orlando Predators, to Arena Bowl XX.

The Imbalance of Power

Paul Hilton "Butch" Davis

Born: 1951
Cleveland Browns: 2001–04
Position: Head Coach
Jersey Number: N/A

SYMPTOMS

Butch Davis grew up in Oklahoma before going on to the University of Arkansas to play football. A knee injury cut his career short but he did earn his degree. After several high school coaching jobs, Davis became the tight ends and receivers coach for Oklahoma State and the defensive line coach for the University of Miami. At both schools he worked under Jimmie Johnson. When Johnson secured the Dallas Cowboys head coaching position, Davis followed him and started as the defensive line coach, before moving up to defensive coordinator. Davis was selected as the Miami Hurricanes head coach in 1995. Credited with rebuilding the Hurricanes program, the Cleveland Browns chose him to replace Chris Palmer in 2001.

In 2001, he turned a 3–13 team into a 7–9 finisher. The following year, the Browns went 9–7 and made the playoffs. Fans expected even more in 2002, but the team tumbled to a 5–11 record and after a dismal start to the 2004 season, Davis was sent packing and replaced by one of his assistants, Terry Robiskie.

Davis's saga in Cleveland was marred by inferior personnel choices and the coach's desire to clean house of players and administrators who had been associated with the Chris Palmer. Dwight Clark, the team's director of football operations, quit in 2002. Ron Wolf, the former general manager who rebuilt the Packers into Super Bowl champions, was brought in after the 2003 season, and lasted only a few months.

After the 2002 season, Davis was undecided about the starting quarterback position and the controversy spilled over into training camp. Kelly Holcomb would ultimately be chosen as the starter based on one playoff game. Davis's draft choices were not successful; Cleveland's number one pick in 2001, Gerard Warren was a major disappointment. William Green, a running back out of Boston College, the 2002 pick, had disciplinary issues in college that followed him during his four-year pro career. Center Jeff Faine was the Browns' first selection in the 2003 draft; he lasted three years and went to New Orleans. In his final draft as head coach, the team selected Kellen Winslow (see page 187).

The pressure undoubtedly got to Davis and some of his decisions have to be attributed to handling the tense situation that losing can bring. Finality was reached after the Browns faced the Bengals in late November. Rumors had surfaced that Davis might not be retained, even though Browns management gave the embattled coach a vote of confidence. The media kept pointing out that the Browns weren't prepared, took silly and costly penalties, and couldn't get plays in on time. The Bengals beat the Browns 58–48. After the loss, Davis sent his wife and eleven-year-old son to Florida to avoid all the attention. Davis finally resigned and indications spread that he might have suffered an emotional breakdown.

Davis came to Cleveland indicating he was going to bring the team a Super Bowl. Instead, he left the team in a super mess.

PATIENT HISTORY

"Butch wears his emotions on his sleeve. When I was the defensive coordinator at Dallas, I was up in the press box and he was on the field. I thought somebody made a mistake, and I yelled at Butch to grab the player. About ten minutes into his tirade, I'm looking at the pictures and we had the wrong guy."
—Dave Wannstedt

"He didn't have a car [in Cleveland] that was in great shape. He's got to drop a new engine in there; the other one wasn't running that smooth. Now he's got to fine tune the engine."
—Corey Fuller, Browns cornerback

"It didn't work out probably because it is a very, very hard job and Butch is a very committed, intense guy. The negativity became very difficult to manage. The pressure on his family was very upsetting for him."
—Randy Lerner, team owner

DIAGNOSIS

When Butch Davis took over the Browns in 2001, optimism was high. Davis was born to coach; he was successful everywhere he had ever been. He was part of, and some say the brains of, the coaching staff that led the Dallas Cowboys to two Super Bowl victories. Davis went on to rebuild the Miami Hurricanes into a national power. He was ready to forge his NFL path—in Cleveland. Davis had a very promising start with the Browns, getting the team to the playoffs in his second year. Ill winds, however, started to blow in off Lake Erie.

First, the Browns' brain trust allowed Davis to seize complete control of the franchise. He was coach and general manager, a combination that most teams found unworkable. Second, Davis used his authority over personnel decisions to cut several veterans in order to relieve salary cap pressure. These players were the ones that helped Cleveland make the playoffs in 2002. Finally, talent evaluation under Davis contributed to lackluster draft picks and a poor defense, the area which was Davis's strong suit.

Davis also had communication and control lapses. His tenure also saw some of the most bizarre events a coach and team would want to endure. Along with the quarterback controversy, and the salary cap purge, the team went through "Bottlegate" in 2001. Fans rained full and empty bottles and cups onto the field after the Browns had a first down at Jacksonville's nine-yard line taken away, despite running a play before the officials reviewed the previous play. Under NFL rules, a challenge must be made before the next play takes place. The incident gave Cleveland a black eye.

In the 2002 season opener, Dwayne Rudd threw his helmet fifteen yards downfield in celebration after he thought he had sacked Kansas City Quarterback Trent Green to end the game. Unfortunately, Green had gotten off a pass, moving the ball to the Cleveland twenty-eight-yard line. Since the game couldn't end on a defensive penalty, Rudd was called for unsportsmanlike conduct, the Chiefs were allowed to kick a field goal, and sent the Browns home as losers.

After owner Al Lerner died in 2002, Butch Davis was without his strongest supporter. Adding all of these problems together, the team eventually quit on the head coach. The media gladly encouraged the revolt between Cleveland fans, players, and the head coach. Davis was not prepared to face the criticism, especially after his early success. The outcome might have been different in another place or at another time, but the need for victories forced Davis out.

SECOND OPINION

Lord Acton, the nineteenth-century British historian, noted that power tends to corrupt and "absolute power corrupts absolutely." Butch Davis's stint in Cleveland proved this axiom. At Miami, Davis was the ultimate authority. Hurricane players didn't have agents or contracts with performance clauses. The NFL was a different story. Many Browns players coached by Davis indicated he wasn't a great communicator and at times was disingenuous. Davis later admitted that he had Browns employees monitor locker room conversations. Without the trust of players, Davis was bound to fail.

The sad part is the Browns had some NFL experienced coaches they could have tapped: San Francisco Offensive Coordinator Marty Mornhinweg, New Orleans Offensive Coordinator Mike McCarthy, Baltimore Defensive Coordinator Marvin Lewis, or Tennessee Defensive Coordinator Gregg Williams. The team was also interested in the Giants Defensive Coordinator John Fox and Offensive Coordinator Sean Payton. True, any one of these coaches might not have succeeded, but none of them would have had to readjust to the NFL.

TREATMENT

An estimated 2.4 million people experience a panic attack each year. Individuals who contend with recurrent panic attacks, have persistent anxiety or fear regarding their panic attacks, and change their behavior in an attempt to avoid further panic attacks, might have panic disorder. The attacks might begin as tightness in the chest, accompanied by shortness of breath or a galloping heartbeat, which sufferers believe are signs of heart attacks and the need to seek immediate treatment.

Researchers believe that possible causes of panic attacks are:

- Triggering of the body's "fight or flight" response without any real threat;
- Fewer than normal serotonin receptors in the brain; or
- Overly sensitive "suffocation alarm systems," which detect a shortage of oxygen even under normal conditions.

Treatments can include pharmacological options, such as serotonin reuptake inhibitors, tricyclic antidepressants, monoamine oxidase inhibitors, or benzodiazepines. Cognitive behavior therapy can also be helpful consisting of panic education, cognitive restructuring, breathing and respiratory control, and exposure therapy. In many cases, a combination of drug and cognitive therapy produces the best outcomes.

INCIDENTAL FINDINGS

After Earl Campbell, the five-foot-eleven, 232-pound Hall of Fame running back, retired from football, he began to suffer from panic disorder that was coupled with agoraphobia (which usually involves the fear of crowds, bridges, or of being outside alone). After seeking professional help, Campbell documented his struggles in a book entitled *The Earl Campbell Story: A Football Great's Battle with Panic Disorder*.

John Madden, the former Oakland Raider coach and CBS analyst, hasn't flown since 1979. He was famous for taking his personal bus to cover games. In the late seventies, he experienced a panic attack on a flight due to claustrophobia (an irrational fear of having no escape or being closed in). Former NFL running back Ricky Williams has suffered from social anxiety and was briefly a spokesperson for Paxil (a selective serotonin reuptake inhibitor).

The Hurricane That Never Made Landfall

Kellen Boswell "K-2" Winslow II

Born: 1983
Cleveland Browns: 2004–08
Position: Tight End
Jersey Number: 80

SYMPTOMS

The 2003 Browns offense wasn't very effective, finishing 29 out of 32 teams and averaging less than 16 points per game. The team needed a player who could make an instant impact. Trading up one spot to number six, Cleveland chose the six-foot-five, 245-pound tight end Kellen Winslow II, who had played his college ball at Miami University. Winslow, a junior, was the highest tight end drafted in almost thirty years. To get the Miami receiver, the Browns traded their second-round pick (thirty-seventh overall) to the Detroit Lions. Browns Coach Butch Davis had recruited Winslow to Miami and Davis was instrumental in bringing him to Cleveland, too.

Winslow's father was a Hall of Famer at the same position, and the Browns hoped that his son could provide similar skills and contributions. Winslow had doubters, though, since he seemed arrogant and unreserved. After a loss to Tennessee in November 2003, the tight end ranted in the locker room about how football was war and players were out to kill him, so he would do the same to them. During the game, he had received an unsportsmanlike conduct penalty for taunting a Tennessee player after leveling him with a hard block in the third quarter. Before the draft, Winslow had shown up late and then fell asleep during a meeting with the Washington Redskins.

The on-field accomplishments of Winslow, however, were without dispute. Winslow was one of the nation's most highly regarded high school all-around players, starring at three positions—receiver, tight end, and defensive end. He continued to impress as a Hurricane All-American, winning the 2003 John Mackey Award as the best collegiate tight end. Draft analysts raved about Winslow's skills of a wide receiver with the stature of a tight end. The team that drafted the star would be adding a dynamic dimension to its passing game.

Cleveland fans could hardly wait to see Winslow in action, but fate interceded. On September 19, 2004, in the second game of his rookie season, with six seconds remaining against the Cowboys, Winslow fractured his fibula all the way through. He underwent surgery, which entailed inserting a plate and screws to aid the healing process. Later it was learned that he also broke his ankle and required additional surgery to stabilize ligaments. Browns fans hoped he would heal in time for the next season.

Unfortunately, while testing out a new motorcycle in May 2005, Winslow crashed the bike and sustained internal injuries and tore the anterior cruciate ligament in his right knee. His season was over, and to further complicate matters, he developed a staph infection during his rehabilitation. Winslow returned to the Browns in 2006, but had issues with the team's coaches and play calling. He did make the Pro Bowl in 2007 after he caught 82 passes for 1,106 yards and 5 touchdowns. Nevertheless, the success of the 2007 season appeared to be an aberration, as Winslow and the rest of the Browns offense declined in 2008. Winslow played just 10 games during 2008 and was traded to the Tampa Bay Buccaneers on February 27, 2009, for a second-round pick in the 2009 NFL Draft and a fifth-round pick in the 2010 NFL Draft. Instead of becoming the next "Wizard of Oz" Newsome, Winslow ended up taking the yellow brick road out of town.

PATIENT HISTORY

"[Detroit] indicated that's who [Winslow II] they were going to take, so that's why the compensation was maybe a little bit higher

than people would have thought. I think that signifies how important Kellen was to us."
—Butch Davis, Browns coach

"With his desire to be great, I think he [Winslow II] can live up to his potential."
—Ozzie Newsome, Hall of Fame tight end

"I feel sorry for any linebacker who is going to have to go up against him this year. But to be honest, I don't think any team's stupid enough to cover him with just one man."
—Jonathan Vilma, University of Miami teammate

DIAGNOSIS

Kellen Winslow was supposed to make a difference. He had a fiery disposition and explosiveness, the likes of which the city hadn't seen since the Cuyahoga River caught fire in 1969. Winslow garnered a national reputation as a college star and a self-described "soldier" on the field. His toughness and passion was the remedy Browns fans yearned for on an uninspired team.

Unfortunately, because of the devastating injuries he suffered in his first two seasons, much of his passion was spent rehabbing his body. By the time Winslow was playing consistently again, he seemed older than a player in his midtwenties. Winslow's performance did not meet the expectations of Browns fans. The tight end's motorcycle injury greatly contributed to fan disappointment because it showed the irresponsible side of an athlete who should have risen to All-Pro status.

SECOND OPINION

Taking a tight end so high in the draft was a bit suspect. After all, Browns quarterbacks were sacked 41 times in 2003. Throwing to any receiver was contingent upon keeping the signal caller in an upright position.

The Browns passed up several good defensive players, including defensive ends Will Smith, Jared Allen, and Shaun Phillips. While the draft wasn't deep in offensive lineman, Jake Scott (guard), Chris Snee (guard), and Max Starks (tackle) were available. Quarterbacks were probably the highlight of the 2004 draft. Eli Manning and Philip Rivers were chosen with the first and fourth picks respectively. Unfortunately for the Browns, Pittsburgh chose Ben Roethlisberger as the eleventh pick in the first round. Matt Shaub went in the third round, a round where Cleveland drafted quarterback Luke McCown.

TREATMENT

The anterior cruciate ligament (ACL) prevents the knee from shifting or rotating too far during athletic activities. Prior to 1970, tearing of the ACL usually signaled the end of the career for a high-level athlete. Due to more research and improved surgical techniques, ACL surgery success rates are as high as 90 percent today, and many athletes can return to play. However, studies do indicate that the post-ACL-surgery performance levels of athletes is statistically less than their preinjury levels. For a further discussion of anterior cruciate ligament treatment, see page 175.

INCIDENTAL FINDINGS

Only three tight ends in the history of the NFL Draft were chosen before the sixth pick in the first round. Billy Cannon, the 1959 Heisman Trophy winner at LSU, was chosen by the Los Angeles Rams as the number one overall pick in the 1960 draft. Cannon, although he played tight end for several years at the pro level, was more of a running back. Cannon opted to play for the rival American Football Conference.

Mike Ditka was chosen by the Chicago Bears as the fifth overall pick in the 1961 draft. The consensus All-American starred at the

University of Pittsburgh. After a twelve-year playing career where he was part of the Dallas Cowboys' 1971 Super Bowl team, Ditka coached the 1985 Chicago Bears to the Super Bowl Championship.

The Denver Broncos chose Riley Odoms as the fifth overall pick in the 1972 draft. He played his entire career for Denver. As a Bronco, Odom went to the Pro Bowl four times.

Not the Center of Attention

LeCharles Vernon Bentley

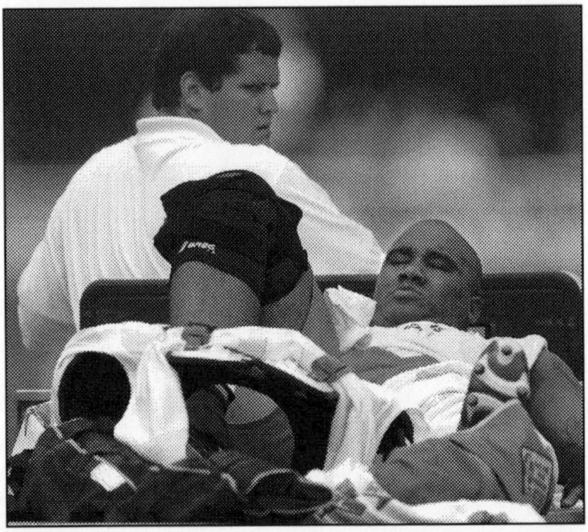

Born: 1979
Cleveland Browns: Never played a regular season game
Position: Offensive Guard / Center
Jersey Number: 65

LeCharles Bentley being carted off the field during training camp, 2006 (Courtesy *Akron Beacon Journal*)

SYMPTOMS

When it comes to parochial schools and football in Northeast Ohio, the names of St. Ignatius and St. Edward are always a part of the conversation. State titles are commonplace and stars from the teams go on to college and even pro careers. LeCharles Bentley, a six-foot-three, 260-pound lineman, played for Ignatius and was an All-Ohio selection in 1997. He became a starting center for the Ohio State Buckeyes and was chosen as the forty-fourth overall pick by the New Orleans Saints in 2002.

Bentley played offensive guard and center for the Saints and was selected to the Pro Bowl at both positions. He became a free agent in 2006 and signed a six-year, $36-million contract with the Browns. In 2005, the Browns' quarterbacks were sacked 46 times, a number near the bottom of the league. Signing Bentley made the experienced and solid lineman a key building block to revitalize the Cleveland offensive line.

On Thursday July 27, 2006, the Browns's first day of training camp, Bentley stepped out on the practice field. Later that day, he was carried off. During a basic running play, Bentley's cleat got caught up in the turf and he tore the patellar tendon in his left knee. His teammates were stunned, but expected the center to make a full recovery.

During rehab at a Browns' facility Bentley contracted a staph infection. The injury and infection required four operations, the latter two to clean out the staph infection, an infection so severe that Bentley almost lost his leg. His tendon was almost destroyed by the infection. Bentley eventually came back for one day of practice, but immediately retired.

Bentley sued the Browns in July 2010, claiming the team convinced him to rehab his knee at their training complex without telling him that other players had contracted staph infections at the same facility. He eventually made an out-of-court settlement with the team. Never one to be the center of attention, all Bentley wanted to do was play center for his hometown Browns. He never got to snap a ball for them.

PATIENT HISTORY

"The initial injury was just a basic patellar tendon rupture. Routine. And as a football player, that's what you sign up for. You sign up to be hurt. That's the nature of the game."
—LeCharles Bentley

"One day I think [Bentley] will be thought of as the best center in the NFL."
—Jim Tressel, former Ohio State coach

"It was a unique circumstance, in terms of him being a local icon, playing at St. Ignatius, Ohio State. It was going to be the trifecta in playing for the Browns. It just didn't work out."
—Phil Savage, Browns general manager

DIAGNOSIS

Bentley had been considered the top free agent available in 2006; he was young, big, strong, tough, and a two-time All-Pro with the New Orleans Saints. Even better for the Browns franchise, he grew up in Cleveland. However, the dream of a long-term anchor in the middle of the offensive line disappeared when LeCharles Bentley was injured. As if the situation weren't bad enough, after the team signed Bentley, the Browns traded center Jeff Faine to the Saints. Faine, a Notre Dame graduate, had been the Browns' first pick in the 2003 draft; three years later he was gone, though the Browns did acquire D'Qwell Jackson as part of the deal. The Browns' salary cap also took a hit because Bentley's paycheck was not insignificant by any means.

Bentley's torn patellar tendon, an injury even worse than an ACL tear, occurred on the first day of full squad contact workouts. A sad and sickening feeling rushed through the fan base; the injury reinforced the feeling that the Browns were jinxed. Bentley wasn't just a good lineman—he was among the best in the NFL. A solid move by the Browns' front office became one with disastrous implications. The repercussions of his injury affected the Browns for the 2006 season, and, ultimately, for several subsequent seasons.

SECOND OPINION

Patellar tendon surgery is usually quite successful. The unfortunate aspect for Bentley was that he also developed a staph infection. (See Jerry Sherk, page 127.) The Browns paid a heavy price, both a salary and a court settlement, to Bentley. It is reasonable to believe that the star could have returned to the field without the additional damage caused by his staph infection.

Cleveland fans would have been happy to see Bentley on the field alongside the Browns' 2007 draft pick, Joe Thomas. A few years later, the Browns chose center Alex Mack, a move needed to fill the void caused by the Bentley injury. If Bentley had recovered, the Browns would have had a very potent offensive line, since Bentley was skilled at the guard position, too.

TREATMENT

The patellar tendon, along with the Achilles tendon, is one of the body's stronger shock absorbers, handling much of the stress applied to the knee by the powerful quadriceps muscle (see medical illustration, page 309). This tendon connects the quadriceps muscle and the kneecap (patella) to the shinbone and allows basic functions such as walking and running. When the tendon ruptures or tears, the knee becomes unstable. A rupture can be diagnosed by an X-ray because the kneecap moves upward toward the hip. A MRI can be used to evaluate partial tears.

A torn patellar tendon is an uncommon sports injury. The force on the tendon is increased significantly when athletes are in a squatted position (that is, when linemen are in a three-point stance). There is some risk of patellar tendon rupture in athletes who already have had an ACL repair on the same leg, especially in those who used the middle third of the patellar tendon to reconstruct the ACL. The use of corticosteroids, either by mouth or by injection, to reduce pain weakens the tendon. The treatment of a patellar tendon rupture is always a broad reconstructive surgery for athletes. Recovery is lengthy, forcing athletes out of action for twelve to eighteen months or more.

In a study entitled "Patellar Tendon Ruptures in National Football League Players," (*American Journal of Sports Medicine* 39, no. 11 (2011): 2436–40) the authors found that from 1994 through 2004, twenty-two players ruptured their patellar tendons and two others had partial tears. Nineteen players (almost 80 percent) returned to their previous level of playing activity. The most important factors in determining whether an athlete would compete again were the number of years a player had been in the league prior to the injury and how early a player was drafted.

INCIDENTAL FINDINGS

LeCharles Bentley has been generous to his high school alma mater, St. Ignatius. He established the Verneda Bentley Endowed Scholarship, named after his mother. The four-year scholarship is presented to an African American or Hispanic freshman from Cleveland who has financial need. The student must maintain a 2.0 GPA as a freshman and 2.5 GPA the remaining years. Also, as part of his settlement with the Browns, the team agreed to provide six annual scholarships to Ignatius students for a twenty-year period.

Currently, Bentley is running the O-Line Performance Academy, the country's first training center designed solely around the needs of offensive linemen. He's received positive endorsements from participants and NFL coaches. The academy is located in Scottsdale, Arizona.

The Sprain's the Same

Daniel Colt McCoy

Born: 1986
Cleveland Browns: 2010–12
Position: Quarterback
Jersey Number: 12

SYMPTOMS

Mike Holmgren signed a contract to become president of the Cleveland Browns on January 5, 2010. Area fans were excited because Holmgren had developed Brett Favre after he came to Green Bay from Atlanta. In his next coaching stop in Seattle, Holmgren made Matt Hasselbeck into a starter. Hasselbeck had been Brett Farve's backup at Green Bay and led Seattle to playoff appearances and one Super Bowl.

On his arrival in Cleveland, Holmgren seemed ready to duplicate his quarterback development magic. The Browns signed Jake Delhomme, traded to get Seneca Wallace, and drafted Colt McCoy as the eighty-fifth pick in the 2010 draft. Colt McCoy had great college credentials; he led the University of Texas to a 12–0 mark in 2009 and had been named Quarterback of the Year and Offensive Player of the Year by the Associated Press. Still, many general managers questioned McCoy's arm strength and were concerned about a shoulder injury he suffered in the first quarter of the national championship game.

With Delhomme slated to start, McCoy could develop over time. Delhomme had several good years as a Carolina Panther, but the quarterback was thirty-five years old and had been 4–7 as starter in 2009, a season where he threw 8 touchdown passes and 18 interceptions. Holmgren believed Delhomme could help the Browns, and since Carolina was picking up a major portion of his contract, the decision was more palatable.

Seneca Wallace, drafted in 2003 in the fourth round by Holmgren, was a reliable backup in Seattle and provided more versatility than Delhomme. In his limited action over several seasons, Wallace had thrown for 25 touchdowns with 14 interceptions. Wallace was capable of stepping in if Delhomme was ineffective.

The Browns started the 2010 season, but their quarterbacks were stopped in their tracks. Delhomme went down in game one with a high ankle sprain, forcing Wallace to take over. Wallace lasted a little over three games before he went down with a high ankle sprain. McCoy, experienced or not, found himself as the Browns' starter.

On October 17, McCoy faced the Pittsburgh Steelers at Heinz Field, beginning a series of five games where the team posted a 2–3 record, including wins over New England and New Orleans and a close loss to the New York Jets in overtime. McCoy threw for 975 yards and 3 touchdowns in the span. As fate would have it, he then suffered a high ankle sprain, too, in a late November game against Jacksonville and was forced out of the lineup. He ended up starting the final three games of the season, all losses. After the end of the 2010 season, McCoy indicated that his shoulder, injured during the national championship game, had been bothering him during his rookie year. He hoped an off-season of recovery and conditioning would allow the injury to heal.

The NFL lockout that shortened the 2011 preseason may have hurt the Cleveland Browns more than any other team in football. Head Coach Eric Mangini had been fired and Pat Shurmur was hired to bring in a new offensive scheme.

McCoy was ordained the starter and the Browns begin the 2011 season at 3–3, but stumbled, winning only one of their next six games and averaging a paltry 13 points per contest over the stretch. Part of the problem stemmed from the fact that McCoy was being sacked almost three times a game, forcing inaccurate throws. Out of the playoff race by late November, the Browns faced the Pittsburgh Steelers in early December. For Cleveland fans, a win against the hated rival would provide some soothing for a dismal year.

The game turned into a defensive struggle, with Pittsburgh protecting a 7–3 lead well into the fourth quarter. With a little under six minutes left, the Browns were inside Steelers territory and faced second and five. McCoy dropped back to pass, was flushed out of the pocket to his left, and as he lofted a pass to Monterio Hardesty, the Cleveland signal caller was struck head on by Steelers linebacker James Harrison. McCoy crumbled to the ground and appeared dazed. Harrison was flagged for roughing the passer, and after a review of the incident, his helmet-to-helmet hit also got him suspended one game by the league. McCoy missed several plays and returned, but ended up throwing an interception that led to a Pittsburgh touchdown two plays later.

Opinions about McCoy's capacity at the time vary. Browns Coach Pat Shurmur said that McCoy did not show any signs of a concussion and was reinserted after being cleared by the medical staff (see concussion assessment, page 201). McCoy's father Brad was not pleased with the coach's decision; he said his son didn't remember anything after the Harrison hit. The following week the Browns confirmed McCoy had suffered a concussion and he didn't appear in the last three games of the 2011 season. The Browns drafted Brandon Weedon in 2012 and dealt McCoy to San Francisco the following year. Another quarterback era in Cleveland took a severe blow.

PATIENT HISTORY

> "I'm very impressed with Colt McCoy and I think he has the skill set, the skill and ability to be a fine player in this league."
> —Pat Shurmur, Browns coach

> "I've thrown with Colt McCoy. He has a strong arm. He's pretty fast. I think he's going to be a good NFL quarterback."
> —Roger Staubach, Hall of Fame quarterback

"Colt really wanted to go to Cleveland. He thinks Mike Holmgren is one of the best quarterback guys."
—Mack Brown, University of Texas head coach

DIAGNOSIS

Three quarterbacks and three high ankle sprains—irony, cruelty, or comedy? During the 2010 season, the Browns shook off a slow start and began to build momentum. The team's play energized a fan base that was badly in need of a shot in the arm following the LeBron James's public departure. The excitement in the air was palpable when the Jets came to town in week nine, but a loss in that game, followed by the loss of third-string quarterback Colt McCoy, transformed the previously momentum-fueled team into one limping away in a walking boot. Three quarterbacks jogged onto the field and three quarterbacks hobbled off the field with the same injury in yet another twist of fate for the new Browns.

SECOND OPINION

The Browns' drafts under the Mike Holmgren regime actually produced some quality players, including Joe Haden, T. J. Ward, and Jordan Cameron. Ultimately, Trent Richardson was dealt to Indianapolis for a first-round choice that was used to draft Johnny Manziel in 2014.

Coaching choices, however, didn't work out as well. Eric Mangini posted two 5–11 records after his New York Jets tenure of 23–25. Pat Shurmur had a 9–23 record with Cleveland over two seasons. Holmgren indicated that the team might have been better off if he took the helm on the sidelines instead of in the front office. Since returning to the league in 1999, the Browns have rarely been competitive. High expectations and high ankle sprains are common; high finishes aren't.

TREATMENT

A high ankle sprain is (see medical illustration, page 313) also known as a syndesmotic sprain, which is a tear of the tough fibrous ligament between the tibia and fibula in the lower shinbone. The strong ligament is above the bump on the inside and outside of the ankle. Rather than rolling and tearing like a typical lateral sprain, the injury occurs with a "plant, twist, and pop" type mechanism, not unlike the ACL.

The ligament is like a tight, strong zipper. When the ankle twists, the middle bone in the ankle (talus) spreads and separates the two shinbones, "unzipping" the ligament from the ankle toward the knee. The higher the ligament tears, the more significant the injury is. The ligament contains a sizable amount of blood vessels and nerve endings, which can result in intense pain and swelling when torn.

According to a recent report in *AAOS Now* (April 2012, pp. 6–7), most NFL physicians

- Manage syndesmotic sprains with no diastasis (separation between the tibia and fibia) using immobilization, usually with a boot;
- Decide if surgery is necessary by using stress radiographs and MRIs; and
- Find that players can generally return to play in a couple of weeks after progressive weight-bearing activity and a functional rehabilitation program.

For nonoperative treatments with rehabilitation, recovery time can take from six to eight weeks, twice as long as a typical ankle sprain. If surgery is required, recovery time can take six months or longer.

Concussion assessment. The sideline assessment of a player who might be concussed similar to the McCoy case is difficult and, at times, can lead to controversy. Concussions can be overlooked easily or routinely underdiagnosed for a number of reasons. First, an athlete might ignore or not report symptoms of a concussion. Second, many injuries present themselves in recognizable ways—broken bones, cuts, and sprains, for example. Brain injuries vary in presentation depending on which part of the brain is injured. Third, there are no imaging or lab tests that can diagnose a brain injury at this time.

Coaches, athletes, trainers, and teammates want a quick, definitive diagnosis. Unfortunately, working to arrive at a diagnosis requires time and careful discernment about how to proceed. The most commonly used tool, the Sideline Assessment of Concussion (SAC) tool (see pages 321–23) takes up to ten to fifteen minutes, at best, to administer and usually requires that a player be removed to a quiet environment for optimal results.

While the SAC is very helpful and provides much information on a possible concussion, the test is not foolproof. The following disclaimer appears on the test instrument:

> This guide is not intended to be a substitute for the clinical judgment of the treating healthcare professional and should be interpreted based on the individual needs of the patient and the specific facts and circumstances presented.

Because concussions are a "silent epidemic" or "invisible injury," returning to play protocols must be addressed carefully.

INCIDENTAL FINDINGS

In many sports, ankle sprains are the number one injury. Included in this list are basketball, softball, soccer, figure skating, cheerleading, gymnastics, and volleyball. In other sports, ankle sprains are the second most common injury. Ankle sprains account for 17 percent of all football related injuries, surpassed only by knee injuries.

Most initial treatments of minimal or moderate ankle sprains follow the RICE (rest, ice, compression, and elevation) protocol. The West Point Strain Grading System is used to determine the severity of the injury. The system uses four factors—tearing, swelling, joint instability, and weight bearing—to aid physicians in determining the extent of the sprain.

That Rundown Feeling

Peyton Hillis

Born: 1986
Cleveland Browns: 2010–11
Position: Running Back
Jersey Number: 40

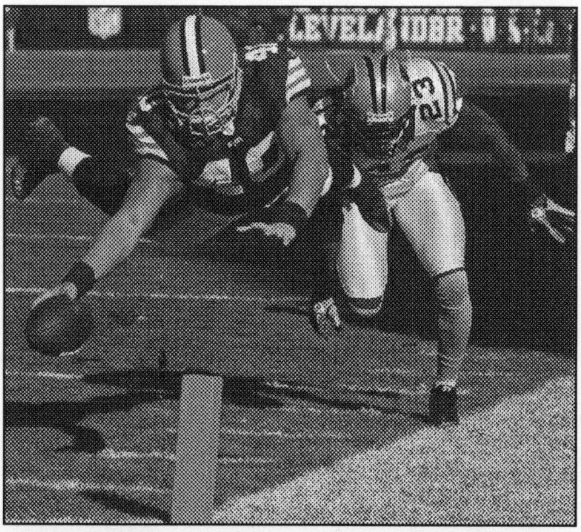

Peyton Hillis stretches for a touchdown against the Carolina Panthers, 2010 (Courtesy *Akron Beacon Journal*)

SYMPTOMS

In many ways, Peyton Hillis's one stellar season with Cleveland was as mythical as his high school mascot, the wampus cat. This creature of folklore has four legs to run on and two more legs to fight off predators. Hillis came to Cleveland in 2010 from Denver in exchange for quarterback Brady Quinn. Hillis, an Arkansas high school star, who went on to play for the University of Arkansas, was selected in the seventh round of the 2008 draft by the Broncos. Hillis was used mostly as a blocker on Razorback teams that featured rushers Felix Jones, a 2008 first-round pick of the Dallas Cowboys, and Darren McFadden, the fourth overall pick by the Oakland Raiders in 2008.

The 2010 season looked promising for the Browns. They had drafted Montario Hardesty in the second round of the 2010 draft, Jerome Harrison was returning after a strong end of the 2009 season, and James Davis, a 2009 pick from Clemson, showed well in training camp. Unfortunately, Hardesty suffered a season-ending injury in the preseason and Harrison was ineffective as a starter and was dealt to Philadelphia in October. Davis was placed on waivers in late October. Hillis took advantage of the situation and became the starter in week three against the Baltimore Ravens, and although the Browns lost, Hillis rushed for 144 yards on 22 carries against one of the better defenses in the league.

Over the course of the 2010 season, Hillis tied a team record (set by Greg Pruitt) with touchdowns in five consecutive games and had 220 yards of total offense in week nine, leading the Browns to a victory over the 6–1 New England Patriots and becoming the first Browns player to be named Offensive Player of the Week since Eric Metcalf in 1992. Despite some late season injuries, Hillis rushed for 1,574 yards and had 477 receiving yards, scoring 13 touchdowns along the way. His gritty and punishing running was a key factor in being voted the cover player for Madden NFL 12, the very popular video game.

Unfortunately, Browns fans saw Hillis on store shelves more than they did on the playing field the following season. Eric Mangini had been fired as head coach and Pat Shurmur introduced the more pass-oriented West Coast offense. A lockout by the NFL owners didn't help the transition to new offensive and defensive schemes. Hillis was also entering the last year of his contract, a saga that was being played out in the local media.

In 2011, Hillis suffered a bout with strep throat and sat out the week three contest against Miami. Some Browns players questioned the running back's commitment and thought his decision had more to do with his contract than his illness. After returning, Hillis strained his hamstring in mid-October against Oakland and sat out several games. Hillis started only nine of sixteen games, during which his average yards per carry dropped from 4.4 to 3.6 and his receptions fell from 61 in 2010 to 22 in 2011.

The Browns chose not to renew Hillis's contract for the 2012 season; he eventually signed on with the Kansas City Chiefs. Many fans suspected the "Madden Curse" was the cause of Hillis's decline. The "Madden Curse" is a superstition that claims that a player who graces the cover of the EA Sports' Madden NFL football video game will subsequently be injured or have an epically bad year. Then again, Hillis's monster season might have been an anomaly and nothing more.

PATIENT HISTORY

> "[Hillis] can play fullback, he can play on special teams, he can play on third down, and that's the guy we were looking for when we made the trade."
> —Eric Mangini, Browns head coach

> "To tell you the truth, I love being a Cleveland Brown. I love being here. I love the city. I love the fans."
> —Peyton Hillis

> "When you're 'injured' and you should be getting treatment, to go do your own thing repeatedly was just disrespectful more than anything to his teammates."
> —Joe Thomas

DIAGNOSIS

Peyton Hillis burst on the scene when Cleveland needed a hero. He was strong and tough, embodying a blue-collar persona that the city could embrace. His rapid rise reached a fever pitch in a football market that lived or died depending on the Browns' final score. His video game cover (he was chosen over the likes of Michael Vick, Aaron Rodgers, and Matt Ryan) topped off an incredible first season with the team.

Storm clouds were brewing on the horizon in 2011, however, as the labor stalemate affected the Browns, who were implementing major changes. The season started in controversy for Hillis and deteriorated from that point on. At the first inklings of Hillis's decline, the media labeled Hillis as yesterday's news and blamed the Browns' front office for inaction. First there was the contract issue. Next, the strep throat incident became a controversy, especially because Hillis's agent had advised his client to sit out the game. Then, a hamstring injury forced Hillis to the bench and left the Browns with little rushing power. Finally, around midseason, a new story broke about Hillis's mystery wedding, which Cleveland fans decided showed a lack of commitment to the team.

When Hillis returned late in 2011, ill will permeated the team's chemistry and the running back was playing out the string. Left with a large void at running back, the team chose a new direction. The Browns traded up in the 2012 draft and selected Trent Richardson from Alabama. Hillis signed a modest, one-year contract with the Kansas City Chiefs.

SECOND OPINION

In November 2011, reports surfaced that teammates had held an intervention with Hillis to address his poor attitude. During 2010, Hillis was said to have been positive and inspirational. Obviously, contract issues played a part in his change of heart. He was scheduled to be paid $550,000 in 2011, even though he finished eleventh in the league—carrying the ball 270 times for 1,177 yards. The NFL labor dispute probably did not help Hillis and he began the 2011 season feeling undervalued.

There wasn't much difference between the 2010 and 2011 Browns, especially on the offensive side of the ball. Even with Hillis's stellar 2010 season, the Browns ranked 31 out of 32 teams in points scored (271). The following year they moved up one ranking to 30, but scored only 218 points. Shurmur's West Coast offense wasn't doing well on the shores of Lake Erie.

TREATMENT

Common symptoms of strep throat, a bacterial infection, include:

- Severe and sudden sore throat without coughing, sneezing, or other cold symptoms.
- Pain or difficulty with swallowing.
- Fever over 101°F (38.3°C).
- Swollen tonsils or lymph nodes.
- White or yellow spots or coating on the throat and tonsils.
- Bright red throat or dark red spots on the roof of the mouth at the back near the throat.

Because these symptoms overlap with other viral infections, strep throat (Group A beta-hemolytic streptococcal—GABHS) is likely overdiagnosed, especially without testing. Even though the rate of identifying GABHS without a throat culture leads to unnecessary prescriptions, only about 25 percent of physicians order the appropriate test. The sheer volume of cases is a factor in simply prescribing antibiotics, but patients also feel more reassured if they receive a prescription from a doctor.

Some of the more difficult decision in sports medicine involve determining if an injured athlete is ready to return to play. Medical professionals face similar decisions in dealing with infections and illnesses. One useful guide is called the "neck check." If an athlete has symptoms that are above the neck (nasal congestion, sniffles, runny nose, sneezing, or sore throat), sporting activity, perhaps at a lesser level, is permitted. If, on the other hand, the symptoms are below the neck (fever, chills, body aches, wheezing, cough, shortness of breath, or stomach pain), the athlete should be held out of play and take time to recuperate. Strep throat is extremely contagious and especially so in closed quarters like locker rooms, therefore, infected individuals should be kept away from other team members.

INCIDENTAL FINDINGS

Perhaps the Madden curse is real or maybe Madden selects players who are gritty, tough, don't give up, and thus are more likely get injured. The following are a few examples of players who graced the cover of Madden NFL and faced adversity the following season.

- Garrison Heart—Broke his ankle and was out for two seasons.
- Daunte Culpepper—Went on to have a disastrous season in 2002, breaking the record for most fumbles in a season.
- Marshall Faulk—A string of bad knee injuries forced him to retire.
- Michael Vick—Suffered a broken fibula after appearing on the cover.
- Donovan McNabb—Tore his ACL and meniscus in his right knee.
- Shaun Alexander—Suffered a foot injury and missed six games.
- Troy Polamalu—Sprained his MCL in the first game of the following season.

Cleveland Cavaliers

1970–present National Basketball Association
Last Championship: None

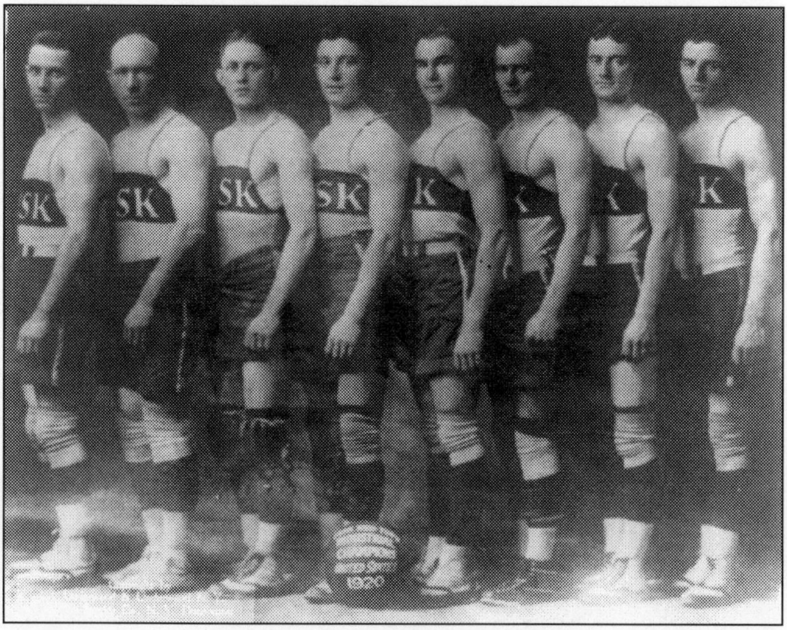

Industrial League basketball teams were sponsored by US industry in the early twentieth century. Pictured are the Fisk Red Tops (sponsored by Fisk Rubber) who played teams from Goodyear and Goodrich of Akron in the summer of 1920 (Library of Congress, Prints & Photographs Division, LC-USZ62-90012)

In 1891, Dr. James Naismith invented the game of basketball in order to provide an activity to fill the gap between football and baseball seasons. The early game had few rules, allowing nine men on each team, which produced a congested court and a large amount of blocking, checking, and obstruction. As the rules were refined, the game caught on, especially at the club and collegiate levels.

Some intercity professional leagues developed after 1910, but the first truly professional league, the American Basketball League, was formed in 1925. Cleveland's entry in the league was named the Rosenblums after the team's owner Max Rosenblum, who owned a local clothing store. The Rosenblums won three championships until economic conditions forced the team to leave the league twelve games into the 1930–31 season. The team continued to play as a touring team during the 1930s.

In 1939, Al Sutphin, who owned the Cleveland franchise in the American Hockey League, worked with owners of the Warren Penns of the National Basketball League to move the team to Cleveland to increase attendance. The Penns became the Cleveland White Horses because Cleveland's White Motor Company bought a large block of seats for the team's games. The experiment didn't work and the team was disbanded following the season. The National Basketball League, which formed in 1937, joined with the Basketball Association of America to form the National Basketball Association in 1949.

Cleveland had a team in the Basketball Association of America for one season (1946–47), the inaugural season of the organization. From the late forties until the early sixties, Cleveland was without a national pro franchise. In 1961, Abe Saperstein, Paul Cohen, and George Steinbrenner formed the American Basketball League. Among the league's founding teams was Steinbrenner's Cleveland Pipers. The squad won the league championship in its first season (1961–62). Following the 1961–62 season, Steinbrenner recruited basketball sensation Jerry Lucas to play for the Pipers with the hopes of becoming an NBA team. The NBA refused to allow the team to join the league, and Steinbrenner disbanded the team before the start of the ABL's second season.

Professional basketball returned to the shores of Lake Erie in 1970. Nick Mileti organized the Cleveland Cavaliers, a professional basketball team that became a member of the NBA. The team's first home was the Cleveland Arena. The Cavaliers moved to the Richfield Coliseum in 1974, and now play home games downtown at Quicken Loans Arena (formerly Gund Arena).

When Clyde Didn't Glide

Walt "Clyde" Frazier Jr.

Born: 1945
Cleveland Cavaliers:
1977–79
Position: Point Guard
Jersey Number: 11

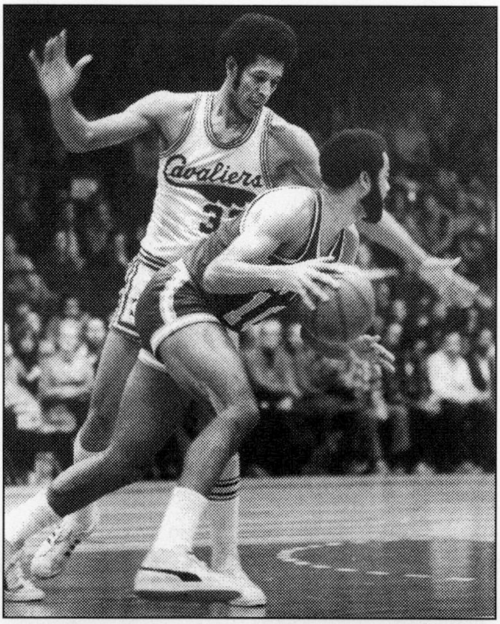

Walt Frazier, as a New York Knick, drives past John Johnson of the Cavaliers, 1971 (*The Cleveland Press* Collection, Cleveland State University, Paul Tepley, photographer)

SYMPTOMS

When Walt "Clyde" Frazier found out he had been traded from the New York Knicks to the Cleveland Cavaliers in 1977, he contemplated not reporting to the team. The Big Apple was what Clyde was all about—leading the high life in the city that never slept and playing hoops at Madison Square Garden. Cleveland was in the wilderness west of the Hudson River and wasn't big enough for Frazier's personality or his Rolls Royce.

The Cavaliers had made the playoffs in the previous two seasons. Perhaps with Frazier onboard, the team might be able to progress further than the first round. Cleveland got Frazier as compensation for the Knicks' free-agent signing of guard Jim Cleamons. Frazier was a seven-time All-Star and had won NBA Championships in 1970 and 1973.

Walt Frazier played high school sports at Atlanta's all-black David Howard High School. He was the quarterback for the football team, a catcher on the baseball team, and a guard on the basketball team. Frazier was offered a football scholarship to the University of Kansas and Indiana University. However, he chose to go to Southern Illinois University, because he wasn't likely to play quarterback for the Jayhawks or Hoosiers due to the racial climate in the early 1960s. At Southern Illinois, Frazier earned Little All-American honors three times. He led the Salukis to the 1967 National Invitational Tournament title and was named the tournament's MVP. The Salukis beat Duke, Rutgers, and Marquette on their way to the championship.

In his first season with the Cavaliers, Frazier played in 51 games and averaged 16.2 points per game, 4.1 rebounds per contest, and 1.5 steals. Frazier's season, however, took a dark twist in a February 20 game against the Bulls. In the third quarter, Frazier severely sprained his left foot and left the game. The point guard would not come back for the rest of the season or the playoffs.

The Cavaliers lost to the New York Knicks in a first-round playoff series while Frazier watched on the sidelines. Still, Frazier's experience and guile was helping the team's chemistry and the coming season might lead to a longer playoff run. Unfortunately, Frazier's time on the court over the next two seasons was as frequent as sunny days in Cleveland during February. Clyde was sighted in uniform fifteen times, reinjuring his foot in training camp and in a November game. The Cavaliers finished the 1978–79 campaign with a record of 30–52 and Coach Bill Fitch stepped down. Stan Albeck came in the following season and the Cavs limped in with a 37–45 record, which ended Albeck's tenure. The Walt Frazier signing ended up costing the team more than points—the team paid Frazier $675,000 over three years for sixty-seven games (Frazier was owed $1.35 million, but the Knicks paid the other half of his salary). The Cavaliers would not finish above .500 again for almost a decade.

PATIENT HISTORY

"I think we got the best player to come out of college this year."
—Dick McGuire, Knicks coach

"He has one of the best reverse dribbles in the world . . . and Frazier is one of the better shooters."
—John Havlicek, Boston Celtics

"I'll be very nervous when I get to Cleveland. It's a new situation, a new team, a new city. I'm 'Cool Clyde,' but I'm not that cool."
—Walt "Clyde" Frazier

DIAGNOSIS

Frazier came to Cleveland late in his career with plenty of injury "baggage." The Cavaliers were at a crossroads; the team was on its way down from "The Miracle of Richfield" years but had not yet reached the lows of the Stepien era. The Cavaliers had lost Jim "The Cat" Cleamons, arguably the emotional leader of the team, and picked up Frazier as compensation. Frazier had gotten rid of the $3,000 mink coat, the 1965 Rolls Royce, and the wide brim hat that earned him his nickname (after Clyde Barrow of Bonnie and Clyde fame). He tried to make a go of it in Cleveland, but he only played sixty-six games in his three seasons. Some fans wondered if he was just picking up a paycheck, but in reality the chronic foot pain was clearly limiting his effectiveness.

Frazier's greatest moment with the Cavaliers came on November 7, 1977, when the Cavaliers played the Knicks; Frazier received a three-minute standing ovation from the Madison Garden crowd. He ultimately led the Cavaliers to a 117–112 victory, scoring 28 points with 8 rebounds, 5 steals, and 4 assists. The remainder of his time in Cleveland, however, was forgettable.

SECOND OPINION

In the end, the Cavaliers paid Walt Frazier about the same amount that Jim Cleamons had asked for. Part of Cleamons' reluctance to stay with the Cavaliers had to do with an issue of deferred compensation. The Knicks were willing to pay the guard up front and Cleamons chose the Big Apple.

The hallmark of the Bill Fitch-coached Cavaliers was their reliance on defense. Cleamons was a big part of that formula; during the guard's last season in Cleveland, the team was second in the league in points allowed. In Frazier's first season, the Cavaliers were fourth best in points allowed. Fitch's last (1978–79) season saw that ranking drop to tenth. Stan Albeck had a different strategy, which resulted in a scoring renaissance (the team was third in the league in points scored per contest), but the defense suffered. The team was nineteenth out of twenty-two teams in points allowed per game.

As Cleamons himself noted, he was a player that did all the little things that helped a team win, but might not show up in the box score. A healthy Frazier would have been a boost to the team. On the other hand, Jim Cleamons was more suited to the Bill Fitch style of play.

TREATMENT

The foot pain that limited Walt Frazier in the twilight of his career with the Cleveland Cavaliers was never well documented, although some reports attributed his limited playing time to a foot fracture. Other reports were inconclusive, but a very common cause of foot pain in athletes is plantar fasciitis (see medical illustration, page 317).

The thick fibrous band of connective tissue that connects the heel bone to the five toes on the bottom of the foot (forming the arch) is the plantar fascia. The tissue is like a small trampoline that functions as a shock absorber when athletes run and jump repetitively. When the band of tissue is overused or overloaded, microscopic tearing ensues. The body heals these microtears with scar tissue. Rather than being a true "itis" (meaning inflammation), the fibrous band becomes stiff and scarred. Over 10 percent of the adult population develops the condition during a lifetime. The symptoms are often worse in the morning or after intense exercise.

A medical practitioner often makes the proper diagnosis after reviewing a patient's medical history and performing a physical exam. When pain persists, an X-ray may show a heel spur, which is a result of the problem, not the cause of the problem. In most cases, if the patient is suffering from plantar fasciitis, the spur can be removed surgically, but the patient will still suffer pain in the foot area.

Nonsurgical treatment has improved dramatically in the last twenty to thirty years with a better understanding of the progression of the injury. Treatment includes rest and heel cord stretching. Medicine for pain or inflammation may be helpful early on, but, if these treatments are not successful, a more aggressive approach needs to be taken.

Aggressive treatments may include deep tissue massage, physical therapy with electrical stimulation, ultrasound treatments, and the use of custom made orthotics (shoe inserts). A night splint for keeping the foot in a stretched position often greatly improves symptoms. If these treatments are ineffective, the next step includes steroid injections, which may provide symptom relief, but over time the injections may weaken tendons and could lead to a rupture of the plantar fascia. Surgery is a last resort and is used much less frequently than in the 1970s and 1980s, due to the success rates of nonsurgical options. Other aggressive treatments that are widely used, especially among professional athletes, are still considered experimental. For example PRP (platelet-rich plasma) injections focus on growth factors essential for healing, which serves to "jump start" the body's natural healing response.

INCIDENTAL FINDINGS

Walt Frazier was the fifth overall pick in the 1967 draft. When the Knicks won the 1973 NBA Championship, Frazier was teamed up with a few other players from that draft. The Knicks had picked Phil

Jackson at number seventeen, and had acquired Earl "The Pearl" Monroe from the Baltimore Bullets, where he had been the overall number two pick in 1967. Another player in that draft class, Pat Riley, played for the Los Angeles Lakers, the team the Knicks beat in the finals.

Phil Jackson won one NBA Championship as a player, but led the Chicago Bulls to six titles and the Lakers to three titles. Pat Riley won two NBA titles as a player and coached the Lakers to four titles and led the Miami Heat to three as head coach and GM. Frazier led his team to two NBA Championships and Monroe was part of one championship team. All four individuals are in the Basketball Hall of Fame. 1967 was a very good year, indeed!

A Quick Study of Knee Troubles

Austin George "Mr. Cavalier" Carr

Born: 1948
Cleveland Cavalier: 1972–80
Position: Shooting Guard
Jersey Number: 22 (1972); 34 (1973–80)

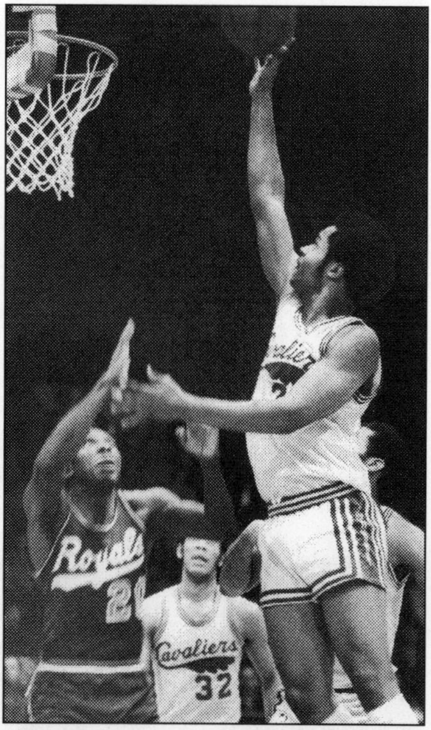

Austin Carr scores over Nate Archibald of the Cincinnati Royals, 1971 (*The Cleveland Press* Collection, Cleveland State University, Paul Tepley, photographer)

SYMPTOMS

Austin Carr was a talented athlete who grew up in Washington, DC. He was named All-City three times during his basketball career at Archbishop Macklin. He also was All-City twice for Macklin's baseball team, playing catcher and batting left-handed. After setting a prep scoring record with 2,124 points and being touted as the greatest schoolboy basketball player in the history of DC, Carr went on to star at Notre Dame. Carr started three years for the Irish varsity, but during his sophomore year he only played sixteen games because he broke the metatarsal bone in his left foot twice.

As a senior in 1971, Carr was a unanimous first team All-American and the Naismith Award winner. During his collegiate career he helped Notre Dame to three straight NCAA tournament appearances and still holds the following tournament records: most points in a single game (61 in 1970), most field goals made in a single game (25 in 1970), best average points per game in the tournament (52.7 in 1970), best career scoring average in tournament (41.3 points per game).

The Cleveland Cavaliers, an expansion team with a 15–67 season record, chose Carr as the first overall draft pick in 1971. Playing in New York's Rucker Summer League prior to his first NBA training camp, Carr cracked a bone in his right foot. Unfortunately, the incident was a precursor of other injuries. After sitting out the first month of his rookie season, Carr refractured the foot in mid-September. Playing in 43 games during his rookie season, the six-foot-four, 200-pound guard averaged 21.2 points per game and was selected to the All-Rookie team. The Cavaliers finished with a record of 23–59.

The Cavaliers added thirty-five-year-old Lenny Wilkens to their roster the following year, and a healthy Austin Carr, with the help of Wilkens, had his best season as a pro, averaging 21.9 points per game and shooting 85.6 percent from the free-throw line. Carr was named to the NBA All-Star team in his third year in the league and seemed positioned to be the Cavaliers' shooting guard for the foreseeable future.

The Cavaliers had put together a young but talented team for the 1974–75 season and hoped to make the playoffs. On December 5, 1974, Carr injured his right knee against Kansas City–Omaha. At first the injury was thought to be a hyperextension, but after an arthrogram, the team discovered Carr had torn ligaments in the knee. Later in December he underwent surgery, ending his season.

Carr returned the next year, averaging 10.1 points per game over 65 games. The Cavaliers made the playoffs, but lost in the Eastern Conference Finals to the Boston Celtics. The "Miracle of Richfield" continued for the next two seasons, sending the Cavs to the playoffs. During the 1978–79 season, Carr played in all 82 games and had his best postinjury season, averaging 17 points per game.

The Cavaliers didn't protect Carr in the 1980 NBA expansion draft and the Dallas Mavericks selected him, but he only played eight games for the team. In November of that year, Carr was traded to the Washington Bullets for future considerations. He ended his NBA career after playing 39 games for the Bullets.

Carr is currently the director of community and business development for the Cavaliers and is a full-time analyst for the Cavaliers Television Network. Fans have become accustomed to his signature calls after Cavaliers' dunks ("Throws the hamma' down"), three-point shots ("From deep in the Q," and after blocks ("Get that weak stuff outta here") and others. His jersey number 34 has been retired by the team.

PATIENT HISTORY

"This is one of the great pure shooters in the country.... He has great touch. He doesn't need a pick. He can free himself for the shot."
—Ray Meyers, legendary DePaul University coach

"When I had two good legs, I could just jump over people or overpower them and do what I wanted to do. Once I had that knee injury, it changed my gait. Consequently, you run differently. Some nights you have good balance and some nights you don't."
—Austin Carr

"What always makes you concerned... is restoring that little spark, a tenth of a second or whatever... that separates a great player like Carr from a good one."
—Dr. Jon Hardacre, Cavaliers' team surgeon

DIAGNOSIS

As the first draft pick in the 1971 NBA Draft, Austin Carr brought something to the Cleveland Cavaliers that any team needed—he knew how to put the ball in the hoop. The Cavs inaugural mark of 15–67 didn't reflect how bad the team's talent was. Despite some bumps and bruises early in his career, during the 1972–73 and 1973–74 seasons Carr averaged 20 points per game. The young guard was showing that his college accomplishments and game were transferable to the NBA.

In 1974, the Cavaliers moved from the decrepit Cleveland Arena to the state-of-the-art Richfield Coliseum. The new surrounding fired up the team and they began to gel under coach Bill Fitch. The added talents of Bingo Smith, Jim Chones, Jim Cleamons, and Campy Russell pointed to a bright, "miraculous" future. Unfortunately, 1974 was also the year that Austin Carr "tore up" his knee.

Carr returned for the 1975–76 season, but he had lost a step and was not a primary scoring option. Still, the team made one of the greatest and most improbable turnarounds in basketball history. After winning the Central Division, the Cavs bowed out in the Eastern Conference Finals against Boston. With a healthy Carr, the final chapter of the "Miracle of Richfield" might have ended with an NBA Championship.

SECOND OPINION

The numbers illustrate how miraculous the Cavaliers 49-win, 1975–76 season was. The team finished seventeenth out of eighteen teams in points scored per game. However, they were second best in the number of points allowed. Three players on the team, Jim Chones, Jim Cleamons, and Jim Brewer all posted their career best points per game average during the miracle season. The 1975–76 Cavs were the exception to the norm. The team did make the playoffs the following two years, but only posted 43 wins each season. The 1978–79 Cavs only won 30 games with many of the players who had been on the 1975–76 team.

TREATMENT

Knee injuries, until recently, were career-threatening, and in most cases career-ending. Surgery was an invasive option, but ACL reconstruction was challenging and the technology to perform such operations was limited. Some doctors considered repair unnecessary. Carr's injury came at a time when strides were being made in reconstructive procedures. Even then, many patients were placed in casts for six weeks, recovery was an extended process, and the likely result was structural degeneration and significant arthritis.

The approach to knee injuries in sports medicine has changed drastically in the last forty years. Arthroscopic procedures (see medical illustration, page 312) with sophisticated instrumentation have allowed for less invasive treatments of ligament injuries, such as those to the anterior cruciate ligament (ACL) and the posterior cruciate ligament (PCL). Athletes who tear cartilage (meniscus) can now have the structure repaired or replaced, rather than simply removed. An athlete with a "blown-out knee" or a knee that is "torn up" faces less tissue trauma and faster recovery. (See Jim Pyne, page 173.)

INCIDENTAL FINDINGS

The Washington, DC area has become a hotbed for college basketball recruiters. The tradition of fine hoops goes back decades. In 1965, Morgan Wooten coached DeMatha Catholic High School to a victory over Kareem Abdul-Jabbar's New York Power Memorial team, which was riding a 71-game unbeaten streak, and put DC-area basketball on the map. Since then, players from the area have played for prominent colleges and universities and have gone on to great NBA careers. Austin Carr is one of eight players from the area who were selected as college players of the year. The other include Elgin Baylor (Seattle, 1958); Adrian Dantley (Notre Dame, 1976); Johnny Dawkins (Duke, 1986); David Robinson (Navy, 1987); Danny Ferry (Duke, 1989); Kevin Durant (Texas, 2007); and Michael Beasley (Kansas State, 2008).

A Basketball Jones Fracture

James Bernett "Sweets" Chones

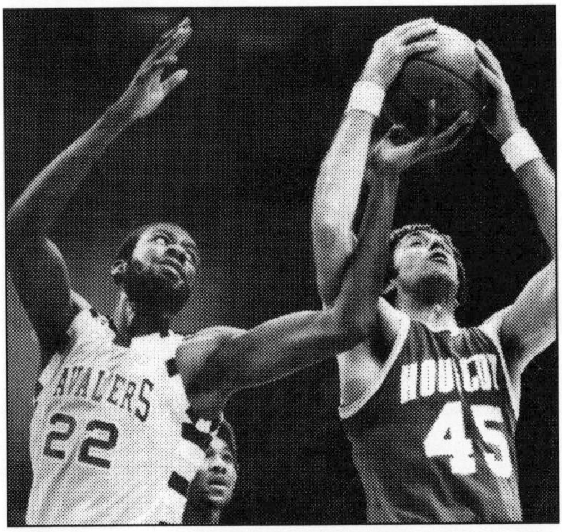

Born: 1949
Cleveland Cavaliers: 1975–79
Position: Center / Power Forward
Jersey Number: 22

Jim Chones fights for a rebound with Rudy Tomjanovich of the Houston Rockets, 1977 (*The Cleveland Press* Collection, Cleveland State University, Paul Tepley, photographer)

SYMPTOMS

Jim Chones grew up poor in Racine, Wisconsin. Many times, his meals consisted of biscuits with sugar and gravy. As a child he picked onions for $.20 a bushel and cut cabbage in freezing cold weather. His parents wanted him to rise above his circumstances and get an education.

Although Chones weighed 155 pounds during his sophomore year, at six foot six he caught the attention of Park High's basketball coaches and became one of the better players in the Wisconsin high school's history. In March of his junior year, he transferred to St. Catherine's and led the team to a 26–0 record and the state championship. He signed to go to Michigan State, but after Coach John Benington died of a heart attack, Chones chose to go to Marquette, in part because his father was gravely ill and the school was closer to home.

Chones had a 50-game career for Marquette over two seasons. As a sophomore in 1971, Chones was part of the 28–1 Marquette team that went to the NCAA Tournament. The following season, Chones led Marquette to a perfect 21–0 start by averaging a team-high 20.5 points and 11.9 rebounds, but his family's economic situation prompted him to sign a five-year, $1.5 million contract with the American Basketball Association's New York Nets and leave Marquette. Chones eventually earned his degree in philosophy from Marquette.

After two seasons in the ABA, the Cavaliers gave up a number one draft pick to obtain the rights for Chones from the Los Angeles Lakers. In his five-year career with Cleveland, Chones averaged 14.3 points and over 9 rebounds per game. During the 1975–76 season, Chones led the Cavaliers into the playoffs and a first round seven-game series win over the favored Washington Bullets. The Boston Celtics stood in the way of the Cavaliers and the NBA Finals.

Fans were primed for a thrilling series and looked forward to the matchup between Chones and Boston's premier big man, Dave Cowens. It would never come to pass; during practice prior to game one of the Eastern Conference Finals, Chones suffered a clean break of the fifth metatarsal on his right foot. He had broken the same foot during the previous season in a January 1975 game against the New York Knicks. Veteran Nate Thurmond tried to fill in for Chones, but the Celtics took the series and went on to win the NBA Championship.

Chones' career with Cleveland ended after the 1978–79 season. He was traded to the Los Angeles Lakers for Dave Robisch, who ended up playing a little over one season with Cleveland, and a future third-round draft choice. Chones won an NBA Championship with the Lakers in 1980. Chones remains active in the Cleveland community and is part of the Cavaliers' radio broadcast team.

PATIENT HISTORY

> "Family is all you really have in life. I never wanted to embarrass my mother or embarrass my father or any of the people I knew who came before me and were part of my life."
> —Jim Chones

> "Jim is the best 6–10 high school player I've ever seen."
> —John McGuires, Chones' high school coach

> "I would say Jim [Chones] is my dart board. I'm not very nice to him, but I think Jimmy knows I'm there if he needs me."
> —Bill Fitch, Cavs coach

DIAGNOSIS

Jim Chones had to be thrilled when Cleveland acquired Nate Thurmond in November 1975. Thurmond helped spell Jim Chones for fifteen to twenty minutes per game and the rotation allowed both players to perform superbly on the court. Chones became an unstoppable offensive force and Thurmond was an immovable defensive object during the "Miracle of Richfield." The team completed the 1975–76 season with 49–33 and with scores of fans screaming for more. The national media started to take notice. The team won a compelling seven-game series over the veteran Washington Bullets, a team that many experts picked to win the NBA Championship. The Cavaliers turned their attention to the Boston Celtics.

Chones' foot injury in practice before the Eastern Conference Finals was one of the cruelest medical blows in Cleveland sports history. Coming on the heels of one of the Northeastern Ohio's greatest basketball highs, the injury cut out the fans' hearts. The loss in the Eastern Conference Finals to the Celtics hurt even more because the Bullets had been considered the biggest obstacle on the road to a championship. The Cavaliers played valiantly against the Celtics, but the team wasn't as effective without Chones. Coach Fitch tried several combinations and gave time to third-string center Luke Witte, an Ohio State Buckeye. With Thurmond fatigued, the Celtics outran the Cavaliers, and the dream was over.

Many thought the Cavaliers would return the next season, but deep down, most Cleveland fans knew the window of opportunity had been forcefully closed. The following year, the team started fast

(8–0) but faded down the stretch to finish at 43–39. The Cavaliers lost in the Eastern Conference first round (2–1) against the Washington Bullets.

The team could have fortified their roster when the NBA merged with the ABA and four of the six ABA teams joined the league (the Denver Nuggets; the Indiana Pacers; the New York, later New Jersey, Nets; and the San Antonio Spurs). However, even though players like Moses Malone, Artis Gilmore, and Maurice Lucas were available, the Cavaliers basically sat out the ABA dispersal draft. Due to their stellar record the previous season, they had the sixteenth pick. The "Miracle" team quickly faded away and the franchise sank back into obscurity.

SECOND OPINION

The 1976–81 drafts played a large role in the Cavaliers' fall from contenders to also-rans. In 1976, the team drafted Chuckie Williams from Kansas State and he lasted one year with the team. In 1977, 1979, and 1981, the Cavaliers did not have a first-round pick. In 1978, the Cavs drafted Mike Mitchell, who lasted three years with the team, and in 1980, Chad Kinch was the team's first-round pick and he had a two-year NBA career. Six years of draft picks didn't provide a genuine NBA starter, except perhaps for Mitchell, who was dealt to San Antonio, ostensibly for cash.

TREATMENT

Many types of fractures occur in the foot but one of the most common in athletes is known as a Jones fracture (see medical illustration, page 315). Sir Robert Jones first described this injury in 1902 in the *Annals of Surgery*. The injury occurs in the fifth metatarsal of the foot, which is involved in 70 percent of all metatarsal fractures. It is differentiated from the more common and much less significant fracture of the bump on the outside of the foot (i.e., the base of the fifth metatarsal). The injury can also be mistaken for a fracture further toward the toes on the outside of the foot, known as a dancer's fracture.

The Jones fracture is diagnosed by X-ray. Acute Jones fractures are repaired with screw fixation of the broken bone using fluoroscopy, especially in athletes, because the fracture does not heal well with rest alone, in part because the fifth metatarsal lies at a watershed (an area of marginal blood flow) between two separate blood supplies. Studies have shown that athletes can return to sports from eight to ten weeks after surgery.

INCIDENTAL FINDINGS

Sir Robert Jones tells of discovery of Jones fracture.

> Some months ago, whilst dancing, I trod on the outer side of my foot, my heel at the moment being off the ground. Something gave way midway down my foot, and I at once suspected a rupture of the peroneus longus tendon. By the help of a friend I managed to walk to my cab, a distance of over 300 or 400 yards. The following morning I carefully examined my foot and discovered that my tendon was intact. There was a slight swelling over the base of the fifth metatarsal bone. I endeavored to obtain crepitus [popping, grating or cracking sensation of joints] and failed. A finger on the spot gave exquisite pain. Body pressure on the toes, even the slightest, was painful; but when the pressure was deviated to the outer side the pain was still greater. Extension of the ankle and flexion of the toes were immediately felt at the base of the fifth metatarsal.
>
> I hobbled down-stairs to my colleague, Dr. David Morgan, and asked him to X-ray my foot. This was done, and the fifth metatarsal was found fractured about three-fourths of an inch from its base." (*Annals of Surgery* 35, no. 6, June 1902: 697–700)

Weak in the Knees but not Heart

Nathaniel "Nate the Great" Thurmond

Born: 1941
Cleveland Cavaliers: 1976–77
Position: Center / Power Forward
Jersey Number: 42

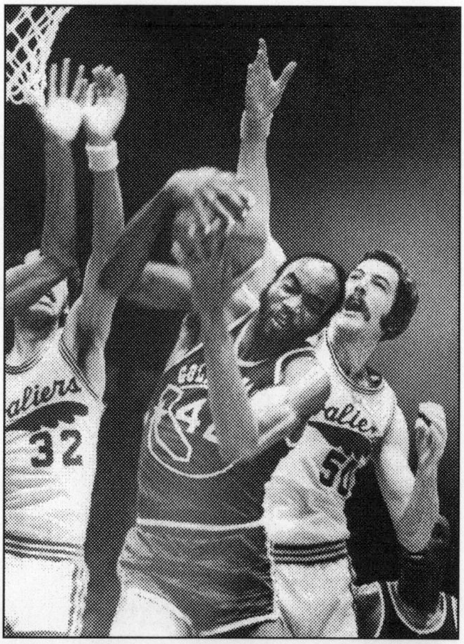

Nate Thurmond, as a Golden State Warrior, battles on the boards against the Cavaliers, 1971 (*The Cleveland Press* Collection, Cleveland State University, Paul Tepley, photographer)

SYMPTOMS

Ohio high school basketball between 1958 and 1959 produced four future Hall of Famers—Jerry Lucas, John Havilicek, Gus Johnson, and Nate Thurmond. Two, Johnson and Thurmond, played together on Akron's Central High School team. With Lucas and Havlicek opting to play for Ohio State after high school, Thurmond chose Bowling Green State University so he'd get ample playing time. Thurmond was a ferocious rebounder at six foot ten, weighing 215 pounds. He averaged 17.0 rebounds and 17.8 points over three varsity seasons, earning All-America honors as a senior in 1963.

Thurmond was chosen as the third overall pick in the 1963 NBA draft by the San Francisco (Golden State) Warriors. He was a seven-time All-Star and a two-time All-NBA Defensive First Team selection. During one season, Thurmond averaged over 20 points and 20 rebounds a game. He was also credited with posting the first official quadruple double while playing for the Chicago Bulls during the 1974–75 season. He scored 22 points, with 14 rebounds, 13 assists, and 12 blocked shots. He career was well-known for battles with the other premier centers in the league at the time, Bill Russell, Kareem Abdul-Jabbar, and Wilt Chamberlain.

Thurmond was traded to Cleveland in late November 1975, along with forward Rowland Garret, for Steve Patterson and rookie Eric Feinstein. At the time, the Cavaliers were last in the Central Division with a record of 6–11. Thurmond's leadership and experience immediately improved the team's chemistry, and he helped lead the Cavaliers to the "Miracle of Richfield" season record of 49–33. The Cavaliers beat the Washington Bullets in the first round of the playoffs, but lost Jim Chones to an injury before the second round series against Boston. Thurmond, who had been coming off the bench, started and faced the Celtics All-Star center Dave Cowens and averaged 10 points a game. However, the Cavs' rotation was impacted and Boston went on to take the series in six games.

Thurmond was a mainstay during the 1975–76 campaign. He would come back the following year, but only play in 49 games due to a knee injury and retire after the season. The Cavaliers did make the 1977 playoffs and Thurmond did his best Willis Reed impression by appearing briefly in game one of the playoffs, which helped inspire his team to victory. However, the Cavs lost to the Bullets and miracles exited the Coliseum.

PATIENT HISTORY

"Nate played me better than anybody. He was tall, had real long arms, and most of all, he was agile and strong."
—Kareem Abdul-Jabbar

"There's no doubt he was one of the best big men to ever put on a pair of tennis shoes. The big fella was first class all the way."
—Austin Carr

"Nate was the catalyst, the man who brought it [Miracle of Richfield] all together. He was the spirit of that club."
—Joe Tait, Cavaliers announcer

DIAGNOSIS

Nate Thurmond took Cleveland fans on a heart-pounding ride, and the fans returned the favor with a show of passion for the team. The "Miracle of Richfield" came at a time when Northeast Ohio was desperate for any good news in a year of Watergate indictments and high unemployment. The team and its fans bonded, raising attendance and the decibel level at the Richfield Coliseum. Thurmond came off the bench and his energy led to impressive scoring spurts for twelve to fifteen minutes per game.

When Chones was injured during practice prior to the 1976 Eastern Conference Finals, the team's rotation suffered. As a result, Thurmond had to play thirty to thirty-five tiring minutes per game. Thurmond's backup Luke Witte, a center out of Ohio State, could only muster 16 points in five games. The Cavaliers finally succumbed to the Celtics in six games. Earlier in his career, Thurmond would have relished the matchup against Dave Cowens, the Celtic's center. With his aching knees and seven-year age difference, Thurmond didn't have the physical presence to stop the Celtic's All-Star.

Even though the "Miracle of Richfield" didn't result in an NBA title, the marvelous run by the team was fantastic. In their prior five seasons in the league, the Cavaliers had finished no higher than third and had averaged 22 games behind the division leader at season's end. The team's ride was special, but the fall was swift, too. Thurmond was gone after two years with "worn out" knees, but his jersey still hangs from the rafters above the team's home court.

SECOND OPINION

The character of Nate Thurmond definitely helped the Cavaliers reach their full potential during the "Miracle of Richfield" season. However, would the aging star have been obtained by the Cavs if they had signed their 1975 second-round draft pick, Dan Roundfield? The Cavaliers were aware that they needed some size up front and they had already taken John Lambert out of USC in the latter stages of the first round. Lambert was a six-foot-ten power forward who primarily came off the bench in his five-plus seasons with the team.

Roundfield opted to sign with the Indiana franchise of the ABA. He had a twelve-year professional career; he was chosen as an All-Star three times when he was a member of the Atlanta Hawks. Roundfield was a consistent force on the court, averaging 14.3 points and 9.2 rebounds a game over his career. The ironic part is that Roundfield opted for the ABA the year prior to the two leagues' merger.

TREATMENT

Knee surgery was never considered minor before the development of arthroscopic procedures, one of the best medical advances of the twentieth century. Prior to "the scope," open surgeries for structural injuries to ligaments and cartilage simply meant a large excision followed by the removal of the torn structures. Recent advances allow surgeons to repair, reconstruct, or replace the injured structures. With the removal approach, athletes lost flexibility, strength, and explosiveness. Athletes simply went as far as they could, as long as they could, until their bodies gave out and forced them into retirement.

INCIDENTAL FINDINGS

Severin Nordentoft (1866–1922) was born in Aarhus, Denmark, and spent most of his life there. A self-made surgeon, he has been recognized recently as the first medical professional in the world to construct and use the arthroscope (a modified endoscope) in a knee joint. The details of his clinical work were outlined in a paper he presented in Berlin in 1912 to the German Society of Surgeons, called "Endoscopy of Closed Cavities by the Means of My Trokart-Endoscope." He is credited with introducing the technique to American practitioners. After Nordentoft's initial groundbreaking work with the arthroscope, he shifted his attention to radiotherapy.

Putting the Wrong Foot Forward

John "Hot Rod" Williams

Born: 1962
Cleveland Cavaliers: 1987–94
Position: Center / Power Forward
Jersey Number: 18

SYMPTOMS

John "Hot Rod" Williams's mother died when he was nine months old and his father did not stay around much longer. He grew up in rural Sorrento, Louisiana, after being adopted by a neighbor, Barbara Coler. She gave him the nickname "Hot Rod" because he made engine noises while he crawled around. Never an outstanding student, Williams attended St. Amant High School and, due to his height, became a basketball star for Coach Tommy Wall's Gators basketball team.

Williams was recruited by Tulane University, even though his academic record (he graduated 181 in a class of 292 students and his combined SAT score was 490) did not seem to meet the school's standards. Stories eventually surfaced that a representative of Tulane had left a shoebox containing $10,000 at Williams's home to help him "decide" to attend Tulane. Williams never fit in socially or academically at Tulane, but he did understand how to play intercollegiate basketball.

During his college career, Williams was named to the first team All-Metro Conference three times, was the Metro Conference Player of the Year in 1984, and was a Metro Conference All-Freshman selection in 1982. He finished his career as the second leading scorer and fourth leading rebounder in Tulane history, with 1,841 points for a 16.0 average per game and 809 rebounds for a 7.0 average per game. He led Tulane to two consecutive NIT appearances, reaching the quarterfinals in 1982.

Williams seemed ready to make the jump to the NBA, but a point-shaving scandal at Tulane led to his indictment on three counts of conspiring to fix basketball games and two counts of sports bribery. The Cavaliers took a chance on Williams by selecting him in the second round of the 1985 draft, knowing he might not be available immediately or at all. Eventually, Williams was found not guilty and joined the Cavaliers for the 1986–87 season.

A vital part of the young Cavaliers, Williams was named to the NBA All-Rookie team along with his teammates, Ron Harper and Brad Daugherty. The following year, the team made the playoffs, with Williams contributing 10.9 points per game and 6.6 rebounds per game. Williams's role was primarily as a sixth man, coming off the bench to provide the team with consistent scoring and rebounding.

After the 1989–90 season, Williams became a free agent and signed an offer sheet from Miami for an estimated $26.5 million over seven years. The Cavaliers matched the offer, making Williams the highest-paid player in the league that year, earning more than New York star Patrick Ewing and the Bulls' Michael Jordan. After the signing, the Cavaliers tried to trade Williams to Seattle, but Hot Rod declined the deal. With his gaudy salary, Williams had to be careful to put the right foot forward on the court. Unfortunately, it was his other foot that became an issue; in November, Williams sprained his left foot. Doctors believed that in driving to the basket Williams might have dislocated his left big toe, but shoved it back into its socket on his next step. However, the action caused the sprain and strained ligaments. Williams missed thirty-seven games. Coupled with Mark Price's knee injury, the Cavaliers ended up with a 33–49 season. The team and Williams rebounded over the next two seasons, making the playoffs, but falling to the Chicago Bulls along the way each time.

After nine seasons in Cleveland, Williams was traded to Phoenix in October 1995 for Antonio Lang, Dan Majerle, and a 1997 first-round draft choice, which was used to pick Brevin Knight. Hot Rod also played briefly with the Dallas Mavericks and ended his career in 2000 with the Boston Celtics.

While not a starter, Williams was the type of player needed to win a championship. He was a consistent scorer and rebounder. His versatility made him a competent backup for any frontcourt position. Williams thought the Cavaliers had the talent to win one or two NBA titles, but a team in Chicago always seemed to be in the way.

PATIENT HISTORY

"John [Williams] has never been the smartest person in the world. He doesn't articulate well. But he says it best about himself. 'Some people are book smart. Some people are smart in other ways. I've been given a talent by the Lord to play basketball. That is my way of being smart.'"
—Joel P. Loeffelholz, Williams's defense attorney

"I wanted to play so much this year [1990–91]. People were saying that John Williams wasn't worth the money, that he wouldn't play hard because he got a big contract. Well, I always play hard. I had worked on the weights this summer and I was ready to have a great season."
—John Williams

"That's the flexibility that he [Williams] gave us. He could play center, forward, small forward, if necessary."
—Lenny Wilkens, Cavaliers coach

DIAGNOSIS

Williams's foot injury turned the 1990–91 season into a frustrating one for area fans. The Cavaliers were in the middle of a great run of success and fans anticipated another matchup with Michael Jordan's Bulls in the playoffs. Williams's injury, along with Mark Price's anterior cruciate ligament (ACL) tear, crippled the Cavaliers and the team limped to a record of 33–49. (The Cavaliers registered 18 of those wins after Williams returned in February.) At first the team thought Williams would be out about four to six weeks, but he was off the court for ten weeks. When he did come back, he was still in some pain, and the team couldn't make the postseason.

SECOND OPINION

Cleveland almost made the playoffs in the 1990–91 season, finishing one spot below the New York Knicks, the eighth-seeded team. The injuries to Williams and Price weren't as damaging to the offense. However, the Cavs' defense suffered in many respects, because without Williams, Cleveland had no backup big man. Rookie Milos Babic at seven feet seemed an option, but he was not a strong inside player. During the 1989–90 season, the Cavs blocked 512 shots and pulled down 3,508 rebounds, of which 1,128 were offensive rebounds. In 1990–91, the team had 450 blocks and 3,310 rebounds, of which 1,011 were offensive rebounds.

Cleveland didn't have a first-round pick in the 1990 draft, having traded the pick to the Clippers as part of the Danny Ferry trade. The team also didn't re-sign "Tree" Rollins as a backup for Brad Daugherty. After Williams's injury, the Cavs didn't sign a free agent who could play the center position. If Williams had returned after six weeks as expected, the Cavs might have overtaken the Knicks and made the playoffs.

TREATMENT

A foot sprain or midfoot sprain is a ligament injury by definition. One specific sprain in the midfoot is a Lisfranc injury. This injury (see medical illustration, page 316) occurs when bones in the midfoot are broken or ligaments that support the midfoot are torn. The Lisfranc joint is found where the long bones of the forefoot (metatarsals) come together with the tarsal bones in the middle of the foot.

Athletes who suffer Lisfranc injuries complain of pain in the midfoot region, and in severe cases, are incapable of putting weight on the foot. Almost twenty percent of Lisfranc injuries are missed on initial evaluation because X-rays are not definitive in showing the injury. A standing x-ray can help in making the diagnosis. MRI or CT scans provide a more definitive answer.

If the ligaments and the bones in the middle of the foot are not injured severely, and bones are not shifted out of their normal positions, nonsurgical treatment can be successful. This usually involves casting and resting the foot for approximately six weeks. If the bones or ligaments are injured, causing them to shift out of their normal positions, surgery is necessary to restore the structure using plates or screws. Postsurgery rehabilitation can take from five to six months.

INCIDENTAL FINDINGS

Jacques Lisfranc (1790–1847) studied at Lyons and Paris and graduated in 1813, after which he served for a short time in the army and then settled in Paris. He sought to reduce operative surgery to mathematical rules, and his name is connected with methods of partial amputation of the foot, of amputation at the wrist, the shoulder joint, and the hip, and with methods of resection of the head of the humerus, for removal of the lower jaw, for excision of the rectum, and for amputation of the neck of the uterus. Lisfranc diagnosed the injury that bears his name after treating cavalry riders that were thrown from their horses, but were dragged along because their feet got caught in their stirrups.

> I can say little more of him than that he was a great drawer of blood and hewer of members. . . . I recollect his regretting the splendid guardsmen of the old Empire—for what ?—because they had such magnificent thighs to amputate. I got along about as far as that with him, when I ceased to be a follower of M. Lisfranc.
>
> —Oliver Wendell Holmes (1809–94), doctor

Back to Square One

Bradley Lee "Brad" or "Big Dukie" Daugherty

Born: 1965
Cleveland Cavaliers: 1987–94
Position: Center
Jersey Number: 43

SYMPTOMS

Brad Daugherty grew up in North Carolina, but didn't play basketball until the tenth grade. His first love was stock cars because his father and grandfather raced. In fact, he wore the number 43 as a pro because he admired NASCAR driver Richard Petty. As Daugherty got taller, the idea of fitting his body into a car speeding around an oval gave way to the reality of using his frame to intimidate scorers on the hardwood. After high school, Daugherty, who had skipped the eighth grade, went to the University of North Carolina as sixteen-year-old basketball prospect. The legendary Dean Smith considered redshirting him a year, but changed his mind. Early in his collegiate career, Daugherty got the opportunity to practice and play alongside Sam Perkins, Matt Doherty, and Michael Jordan.

On the day of the 1986 draft, Daugherty appeared to be headed to Philadelphia, the team that held the first pick. The Cavs changed the outcome by trading Roy Hinson and cash to the 76ers. Daugherty, only twenty years old, was now a Cavalier. Fans weren't thrilled with the pick; Daugherty was considered by some as too soft and not able to take the banging in the NBA. Daugherty started 80 games in his rookie season and averaged almost 16 points per game, making the All-Rookie team.

Daugherty became a consistent scorer and rebounder for the Cavs and the team made the playoffs in six of the eight seasons he played. He averaged 19 points and 10 rebounds in the postseason. Daugherty was also a five-time All-Star. When Daugherty was out of the lineup, the team felt it. During the 1989–90 season due to an operation to relieve swelling between the third and fourth toe of his right foot, he missed 41 games and the team won only 42 games, as opposed to 57 the previous year.

On February 17, 1994, against the Knicks, Daugherty began to experience lower back pain. He was forced to the sidelines and fans hoped rest would be all the twenty-eight-year-old needed. However, in early March, the team announced that Daugherty had a herniated lumbar disk, a career-threatening injury (see medical illustration, page 302). At first the team was optimistic, indicating that surgery might not be necessary. Daugherty ultimately missed the last 29 games of the regular season. The Daugherty-less Cavaliers made the playoffs, but were trounced in the first round by Chicago.

After months of rehabilitation, the Cavs started the next season without their star center. In December, Daugherty realized that the only chance he had to come back was to have surgery to repair the two herniated discs, which were causing weakness (mild paralysis) in his legs. After surgery, Daugherty tried to play again, but he never suited up for a game and retired in June 1996.

Daugherty would have had many more seasons as a Cavalier. The loss of his presence prompted the organization to draft a few big men and ultimately sign Shawn Kemp. With Daugherty around, the team might have been able to pick up a premier guard in free agency, a position they desperately needed.

PATIENT HISTORY

"He seems to be the difference. Without Brad [Daugherty], Carolina wasn't big. They were searching. They weren't a team to be reckoned with. Now they're as good as anybody."
—Jim Boeheim, Syracuse head coach

"The feeling on our staff is that the Eastern Conference is much bigger than in the past, and you have to get big people to compete with Boston, New York, and Atlanta. We felt he [Daugherty] was the best player available and the best big man available."
—Thaxter Trafton, Cavaliers president

"I don't know if I'll ever play again. I want to give myself a chance to play, so I am going ahead with this [back operation] and pointing toward next season."
—Brad Daugherty

DIAGNOSIS

Getting Brad Daugherty in the 1986 draft was a great coup for the Cavaliers. He developed nicely as a dominant inside force on a team that had good perimeter-shooting pieces. Despite the fact that the late 1980s and early 1990s Cavaliers had their share of disappointments, expectations were still high that Daugherty would help carry the team to great heights as he continued to develop. However, the team never reached the expectations of the fans and media. Two things interrupted the development of a dynasty. First, the Cavaliers could not find a way to get past Michael Jordan and the Chicago Bulls. Second, the centerpiece of the franchise was gone just as he should have been entering his prime.

SECOND OPINION

The Cleveland fans' negative reaction to the selection of Brad Daugherty has to be viewed in relationship to the 1984 draft trade for Melvin Turpin. If Turpin had succeeded, Daugherty might not have been chosen in 1986. Turpin, however, wasn't a favorite of George Karl because the new Cavs' coach didn't think the former Kentucky center was dedicated to the game. Turpin's nickname "Dinner Bell" might have portended the center's attitude, one that kept him from trying out for the Olympics due to his lack of physical fitness at the time.

The Cavs had a few other big men, including Mark West, who was traded to Phoenix in 1988 along with Kevin Johnson. Charles Oakley was ever so briefly a member of the Cavs until he was swapped on draft day in 1985 to the Chicago Bulls for Keith Lee, another enigmatic big man that didn't last long in the NBA. Oakley helped the Bulls eliminate the Cavs from the 1988 playoffs. He was then traded to the New York Knicks in a deal that brought "Medical" Bill Cartwright to the Bulls, a move that helped the Bulls to the NBA Championship a few years later.

TREATMENT

The intervertebral disc is an oval-shaped shock absorber located above and below each bony vertebra. A tough, thick covering, known as an annulus fibrosis surrounds the disc. As athletes load this disc and rotate repeatedly, the covering can wear out or rupture, causing pain, nerve injury, and arthritis around the joints in the spine. Athletes seem to be more prone to degenerative disk disease than non-athletes.

Intervertebral disc herniations are of four types.

- Protrusion—slight disc deformity without rupturing
- Prolapse—inner part of the disc (nucleus pulposus) has lapsed through all but the outermost layers (annulus fibrosus) of the disc
- Extrusion—the inner part of the disc has moved into the spinal canal
- Sequestered—the inner part of the disc separates and becomes a free-floating fragment.

Nonsurgical treatment for chronic lower back pain can include rest, the use of anti-inflammatory medications, and rehabilitation, including extension exercises. As pain is lessened, increased activity that strengthens the lumbar muscles is called for. If the pain persists, microdisectomy (removal of herniated disc material) or, more recently, lumbar disc replacement surgery can be performed.

Many athletes return to sports following surgery. However, when the discs above and below a single vertebrae require surgery (two-level injury), the risk of instability increases and return to athletic activity is much more difficult.

(Some information for this section was adopted from *The Professional Journal for Athletic Trainers and Therapists* (March 1999): 27–31 and *Seminars in Spine Surgery* (2010): 206–9.)

INCIDENTAL FINDINGS

Brad Daugherty is among several Tar Heels who have been selected to participate in the NBA All-Star Game. Others include: Vince Carter (2000, 2001); Billy Cunningham (1969, 1970, 1971, 1972); Walter Davis (1978, 1979, 1980, 1981, 1984, 1987); Bobby Jones (1977, 1978, 1981, 1982); Michael Jordan (1985, 1986, 1987, 1988, 1989, 1990, 1991, 1992, 1993, 1996, 1997, 1998); Bob McAdoo (1974, 1975, 1976, 1977, 1978); Charlie Scott (1973, 1974, 1975); Lee Shaffer (1963); Jerry Stackhouse (2000, 2001); Rasheed Wallace (2000, 2001).

A Price on His Head

William Mark Price

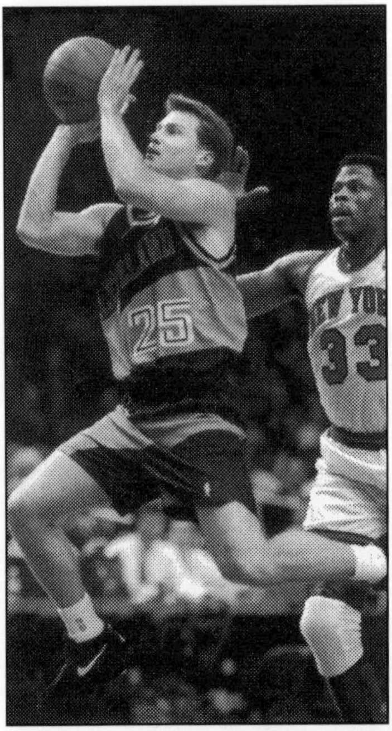

Born: 1964
Cleveland Cavaliers: 1987–94
Position: Point Guard
Jersey Number: 25

Mark Price drives past Patrick Ewing of the New York Knicks, 1996 (Courtesy *Akron Beacon Journal*)

SYMPTOMS

Basketball genes run throughout Mark Price's family. His father Denny played college ball and went on to a career in coaching. Mark's brother Brent had a nine-year career in the NBA. Hudson Price, Mark's son, is a six-foot-six shooting guard and Josh Price, Mark's younger son, plays the sport, too.

Basketball smarts were also a given for the Price family. Mark Price was always considered too small to have a future at the pro level. However, he made up for his size by perfecting his shooting and team leadership skills. In high school during the 1982 Oklahoma state semifinal, Price poured in 42 points (tying the scoring record his father set in 1955) and tossed in 35 more points in the championship game, though his team was defeated. Passed up by many prominent NCAA Division I schools, Price ended up at Georgia Tech, a team that was 14–40 in the two seasons before the guard came to campus.

During Price's career with the Rambling Wreck, Tech posted an 85–41 record, went to the NIT in 1984, and played in the "Big Dance" in 1985 and 1986. Price was named the Most Outstanding Player in the 1985 ACC Tournament in Atlanta, leading Tech to its first ACC Basketball Championship.

Price was selected twenty-fifth overall by the Dallas Mavericks in the 1986 NBA draft and immediately traded to Cleveland for its a second-round pick in 1989. Cleveland also chose Brad Daugherty and Ron Harper in the same draft, making it arguably the best draft in the team's history.

By 1988–89 season, the Cavaliers were contenders for a NBA crown. In late February, they had posted a league-leading record of 41–12. The Detroit Pistons, with the second-best record (36–15), came to Cleveland on February 28 to battle the Cavs. During the game, Price suffered a mild concussion after getting hit by Rick Mahorn's elbow as the Detroit forward set a screen. Price finished the game, but ended up sitting out the next two contests. Mahorn was eventually fined by the league for his action.

In April, the Pistons came back to Cleveland, but this time they had the best record in the league. During the contest, which the Pistons won easily, Price suffered a strained groin injury. Fans were beginning to ask if the February incident had affected the Cavs' psyche, since the team's torrid pace had slowed considerably. The team denied the implications and looked forward to the playoffs and facing the Chicago Bulls and Michael Jordan in the first round.

Unfortunately, Price missed the first playoff game due to his injury, a game that the Bulls won. The five-game series came down to the final game in Cleveland and fans thought the Cavs' regular season 6–0 record against Jordan's team would provide the impetus for a series win. With under four seconds to go Cleveland led 100–99, but

Michael Jordan hit "The Shot" (a moment in Cleveland that has become as infamous as "The Drive" and "The Fumble") to give the Bulls the victory. The following year, the Cavs made the playoffs but lost in the first round to the Philadelphia 76ers.

In the sixteenth game of the 1992–93 season, Price tore the anterior cruciate ligament in his left knee. At the time the team was 9–7. Without Price, the team went 24–42 and missed the playoffs. During a three-season span, starting with the 1990 season, the Cavs had a winning percentage of .625 with Price in the lineup and a winning percentage of .350 when he was unavailable.

Price was a four-time All-Star during his nine-year career in Cleveland and the team went to the playoffs seven times. Due to Price's three-point accuracy and superb free-throw percentage, the Cavs' guard is credited with a move called "splitting the double-team" on a standard offensive play called the pick-and-roll. (An offensive play where a player without the ball sets a screen for his teammate with the ball and then cuts or "rolls" to the basket. He then receives a pass and uses the open lane to the basket for an easy lay-up.) Price was quick enough to dribble between the two opposing defenders and drive to the basket. If the team chose not to double-team Price, he could hit three-point shots consistently or drive against a much slower player who would be forced to foul the Cleveland guard.

In 1996, the Cavaliers traded Mark Price to the Washington Bullets for their top draft pick. The Cavaliers chose Vitaly Potapenko from Wright State with that pick (twelfth overall). Potapenko spent two years in Cleveland and had a journeyman career with several other teams. When Cleveland traded Potapenko, Cleveland received Andrew DeClercq and a first-round pick that was used to select Andre Miller.

During the 1988–89 season, Price became the third player to shoot at least 40 percent from three-point range, at least 50 percent from the field, and at least 90 percent from the free-throw line. Stature was never an issue when it came to Price's talent. Mark Price's number was retired by the Cavaliers in 1999.

PATIENT HISTORY

"Mark's only problem is that every church in Atlanta wants him to come sing in its choir. The kid's a trip. The first time I saw him singing on TV, I flipped."
—Bobby Cremins, college coach

"Mark really revolutionized the way that people attack the screen and roll. To me, he was the first guy in the NBA who really split the screen and roll.... You watch an NBA game now and almost everybody does that. Mark was a pioneer in that regard."
—Steve Kerr, former player

"He's our quarterback and when you play against a team like Boston, Chicago, or Portland—all the top teams in the league—to compete consistently you have to have a player like that."
—Lenny Wilkens, Basketball Hall of Famer

DIAGNOSIS

The infamous "blow to the head"administered by Rick Mahorn, the leader of Detroit's "Bad Boys," changed the direction of the Cleveland Cavaliers franchise. Coach Lenny Wilkens had always stressed great timing and rhythm, in stark contrast to Detroit Coach Chuck Daly's "trench warfare," which included hand-to-hand combat. Mark Price was a casualty in the battle. The Price incident was Mahorn's third strike that year, having been fined twice previously for his rough play. Mahorn infamously had said, "I'll play, I'll help us win, if it kills me. If it kills you" (*Sports Illustrated*, April 10, 1989). One Cleveland fan mailed a death threat to Daly, which spurred an FBI investigation.

With Price's inconsistent play, the team lost its mojo. The Cavaliers were much better than the Chicago Bulls in the regular season and should have dispatched the "Jordanaires" with relative ease. After the season, the Cavaliers front office panicked, trading Ron Harper for Danny Ferry. In the late 1980s, basketball great Magic Johnson had labeled the Cavaliers the "team of the nineties," but Chicago ended up earning that mantle.

SECOND OPINION

Mark Price was the second leading scorer in games four and five against the Bulls in the 1989 first-round playoffs. However, the Cavaliers could not contain Michael Jordan, who averaged 39.8 points per game in the series. In game five, Jordan poured in 44 points.

The Ron Harper trade, along with the selection of John Morton in the 1989 NBA draft, didn't help the Cavaliers. They were left with a void at the shooting guard position. Unfortunately, the price for Danny Ferry was too high, costing draft picks and leaving little room for free agent signings.

TREATMENT

Sports-induced concussions or traumatic brain injuries (TBI) (see medical illustration, page 295) are very hard to diagnose and treat. Athletes often return to play after suffering a concussion, which can affect performance on the field. Symptoms associated with brain injuries can last from days to years. The symptoms include, but are not limited to, headaches, slow reaction time, the inability to sleep, becoming fatigued easily, dizziness, and balance issues. Visual disturbances, such as blurred or double vision, are also associated with traumatic brain injuries. Mood swings are common.

The onset of symptoms appears differently in different athletes, depending on what part of the brain is affected.

- Occipital lobe—changes of visual acuity such as double vision or blurred vision.
- Temporal lobe—houses thinking, reasoning, and memory functions.
- The cerebellum—controls balance and coordination, and dizziness and balance problems are associated with some concussions.

- The frontal lobe—where most emotional symptoms originate.

Athletes may have difficulty controlling their emotions and will exhibit emotional extremes shortly after suffering a concussion. There are no objective tests available to help identify or track the emotional symptoms of a brain injury.

One of the more vexing aspects in recovering from traumatic brain injuries is Post-concussion Syndrome (PCS). PCS is recognized when concussion symptoms persist at least three weeks after the injury. Some statistics show that nearly one-third of athletes with concussions experience PCS. Symptoms can be put into four categories:

- Emotional issues: sadness, anxiety, irritability, and depression.
- Somatic (bodily symptoms) issues: headaches, vision problems, balance problems, light sensitivity, and chronic nausea.
- Sleep issues: insomnia and hypersomnia
- Cognitive issues: attention problems, memory loss, chronic fatigue, feeling "foggy" or slowed down.

These symptoms can last for weeks, months, or even years, and some can become permanent.

Most people with Post-concussion Syndrome are able to recover with rest and reducing or eliminating stressful activities. For those with recurring headaches, migraine or pain medications may be prescribed. Antidepressants and psychotherapy may be recommended for individuals facing psychological problems.

INCIDENTAL FINDINGS

The National Basketball Association has recently developed a return-to-participation protocol for concussions.

- The return-to-participation protocol involves several steps of increasing exertion—from a stationary bike, to jogging, to agility work, to noncontact team drills.

- With each step, a player must be symptom free to move to the next step. If a player is not symptom free after a step, he stops until he is symptom free and begins again at the previous step of the protocol (i.e., the last step he passed without any symptoms).
- While the final return-to-participation decision is to be made by the player's team physician, the team physician must discuss the return-to-participation process and decision with the Director of the NBA's Concussion Program prior to the player being cleared for full participation in NBA Basketball.
- It's important to note that there is no time frame to complete the protocol. Each injury and player is different and recovery time can vary in each case.

Demonized and Distraught

Daniel John Willard "Danny" Ferry

Born: 1966
Cleveland Cavaliers: 1990–99
Position: Power Forward /
Small Forward
Jersey Number: 35

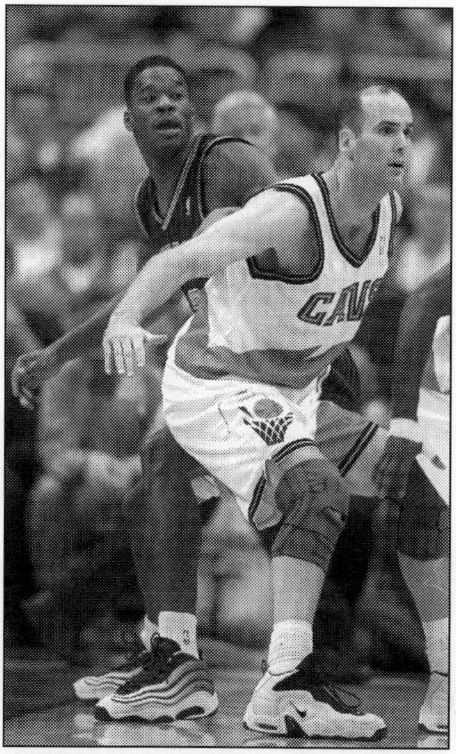

Danny Ferry, with knee braces, battles against the Pacers, 1999 (Courtesy *Akron Beacon Journal*)

SYMPTOMS

Danny Ferry had the perfect pedigree to be an NBA superstar. His father Bob played in the NBA for nine seasons, five of them for the Baltimore Bullets. After retiring from the game, Bob Ferry was a two-time NBA Executive of the Year during his eighteen-year tenure as general manager of the Baltimore and Washington Bullets. Danny Ferry attended famed DeMatha Catholic High School and was named high school player of the year by *Parade* magazine. He went on to perennial college power Duke University and was chosen as National Player of the Year in 1989. He was considered a can't-miss NBA star.

Ferry was selected as the second overall pick in the 1989 draft by the Los Angeles Clippers, but opted instead to play hoops in Italy for Il Messaggero Roma for $2 million. On Friday, February 23, 1990, the Los Angeles Clippers traded the rights to Danny Ferry, along with Reggie Williams, to the Cleveland Cavaliers for Ron Harper and three draft picks, two first rounders and a second rounder. Cavs' General Manager Wayne Embry considered Ferry to be as talented as Larry Bird or David Robinson, but fans were stunned by the move. Ferry signed a ten-year, $36-million contract with the Cavs.

Although the Cavaliers had exceptional seasons while Ferry was on the roster, Ferry never became a superstar at the pro level. In his first six seasons, he only started 11 games. His best scoring season was the 1995–96 season, when he averaged over 13 points a game. If Ferry had blossomed as hoped, the Cavs could have made a run at an NBA Championship since they had a talented nucleus of players. Ferry became a free agent in 2000 and signed with the San Antonio Spurs.

When Ferry initially reported to Cleveland, he was sidelined with tendinitis of the left knee. Playing on a part-time basis, Ferry struggled. His father thought he had changed his game because he was primarily a shooter and needed to adjust his moves to the new environment. What Cleveland fans found out was Ferry had seen his best days as a Blue Devil. Ferry's nagging injuries, his salary, and the lost draft picks were a burden the team couldn't overcome.

Following again in the footsteps of his father, Ferry had a second career in Cleveland as the general manager for the Cavaliers during the first LeBron James era. He made several moves to bolster the team's chances of winning an NBA crown, but when James took his game to Miami in 2010, Ferry resigned. In 2012, Ferry became the general manager of the Atlanta Hawks.

PATIENT HISTORY

"At fifteen he had the basketball mind of a thirty-year-old, not to mention the know-how to execute picks, screens, and body slams."
—Mike Brey, Notre Dame head coach

"Boston waited a year for Larry Bird. San Antonio waited two years for David Robinson. You will see. Danny Ferry will be well worth the wait."
—Wayne Embry, Cavaliers general manager

"I can't wait until he gets here. In college, he was a very good player who made people around him very effective. And he took the big shots and made them."
—Lenny Wilkens, Cavaliers coach

DIAGNOSIS

The Ferry era was a long, painful chapter in Cleveland sports history. Ferry was a nice guy and he worked hard, but his physical limitations were exposed at the pro level. After ten years, Cleveland fans saw a "can't miss" prospect turn into a "can't make" disaster. With Mark Price, Brad Daugherty, Larry Nance, and "Hot Rod" Williams on the roster, Ferry was supposed to be the final ingredient to bring championships to Cleveland.

Further, many fans thought that the Cavs shouldn't have traded Ron Harper, who had been averaging almost 20 points per game. Meanwhile, Ferry struggled to meet expectations. He averaged only 8 points per game in his ten years with Cleveland. The Danny Ferry trade was a "lose-lose" deal for both teams; Harper never panned out for the Clippers. Ironically, as part-time players near the end of their careers, Ferry and Harper won NBA Championships (Harper with the Lakers and Ferry with the Spurs).

The role of Ferry's knee injury may not explain the whole story, but the injury didn't help. David Falk, the agent who represented Ferry, warned future NBA players to reconsider playing overseas. He contended that Ferry's one-year Italian career was spent on antiquated and hard playing surfaces, with inadequate medical care, and with long practices that damaged the Duke player's knees. Cleveland fans just knew it didn't add up to an NBA crown.

SECOND OPINION

Team chemistry is a much-discussed topic. When players fit well together the sum of the parts usually exceeds the players individually. Before Danny Ferry arrived in Cleveland, the Cavaliers had a young, but talented group. Finding the right small forward to complete the puzzle was a prime concern of management.

The Cavaliers drafted John Morton out of Seton Hall in the 1989 first round and Chucky Brown out of North Carolina State in round two. The Morton pick was probably driven by the fact that Ron Harper was traded to bring Ferry to Cleveland. Morton was only a third team All-Big East selection; his NBA career was brief and unheralded. Chucky Brown had a journeyman NBA career playing for twelve teams.

Ron Harper had his best seasons with Cleveland. Perhaps his game just fit well with his teammates. Instead of Ferry, would the Cavaliers have won an NBA Championship if they had traded up in the draft and landed either Sean Elliot or Glen Rice?

TREATMENT

One of the more common causes of chronic knee pain in sports like basketball and volleyball is patellar tendonitis, more commonly known as jumper's knee (see medical illustration, page 310). The ailment is a classic overuse injury resulting from the continual stress put on the large shock-absorbing patellar tendon, which is located below the knee. Initial inflammation, when not properly treated, can result in the development of scar tissue in the tendon in six to eight weeks. At this point, players experience chronic stiffness and pain (tendonitis), which can limit their performance.

A primary treatment to improve elasticity and function of the tendon centers on increasing blood flow (neovascularization) to the affected area. This can be done through deep tissue massage, physical therapy (ultrasound and muscle stimulation), and more recently platelet rich plasma therapy (PRP). Surgery is usually a last resort treatment. Even with treatment, some athletes never regain their preinjury performance levels.

INCIDENTAL FINDINGS

While playing overseas, Ferry showed signs of tendinitis in his left knee, which required regular treatments. Obviously, Ferry had played a great deal of basketball growing up. One study indicates

> that jump performance, as measured by height, is not affected by JK [jumper's knee]. Therefore, just because athletes can still perform, it does not necessarily mean that their condition is minor or not affecting them in another way. Kinematic results show that to maintain jump performance compensations at other joints occur, especially at the hip and ankle. This indicates that special attention should be paid to flexibility and strengthening of the hip and ankle in those with JK because they are being used more. (Julie A. Siegmund, Kellie C. Huxel, and C. Buz Swanik, "Compensatory Mechanisms in Basketball Players with Jumper's Knee," *Journal of Sport Rehabilitation* 17 (2008): 358–71)

Italy has a strong history of basketball dating back to the early 1900s. The following excerpt describes the results from the Inter-Allied Games, which were held in Paris June 22 through July 6, 1919.

The Europeans proved superior in soccer, the sport so popular on the Continent, the United States quite as decisively showed the way in Basketball to Italy and France, the only other entries. Since this game is one of the most popular in America but almost unknown in Europe, the one-sided scores by which the United States won both games from their sports-manlike but less practised opponents were not surprising....

The first game on 26 June resulted in an easy victory for the United States over the Italian quintette. The latter was the first team ever organized in this sport in Italy and it had enjoyed little opportunity for training. The Americans won by a score of 55 to 17 and used substitutes in the second half. Their teamwork, short passing and condition stood out in contrast to the losers who tried disastrous long passes and were weak on scoring. Brennan was the main cog in the mechanism of the winning five, scoring six field goals. The players of both nations were as follows: United States—Ruddiger (R.F.), Greene (L.F.), Brennan (C.), Pelletier (R.G.), Friedman (L.G.), substitutes, Kewallis, May and Brown. Italy—Sessa (R.F.), Baccarini (L.F.), H. Muggiani (G.), M. Muggiani (R.G.), Pecelle (L.G.).

Italy defeated France 15 to 11 on 28 June. This game was exciting throughout, the play at times being excellent. France led at the end of the second half 6 to 5, but Se[ss]a, starring for Italy, shot his team into victory in the final period with 4 successive baskets from the field and one foul goal. Because of unfamiliarity with the rules, more fouls were called in this contest than in either of the other two. As the low scores indicate, both teams were weak on offensive and often missed easy baskets. The players were as follows : France—Bagay (R.F.), Aube (L.F.), Chauvet (C.), Aguillaume (R.G.), Turaglie (L.G.); substitute, Maurier. Italy—Sessa (R.F.), Baccarini (L.F.), H. Muggiani (C.), Pecollo (R.G.), Bagnoli (L.G.).

The final game on 29 June was won by the United States from France, 93 to 8. The winners went at top speed all the way and scored at will. Brennan was again the mainstay with sixteen goals. He seldom lost the tipoff and usually started the ball towards another score. The forwards, Ruddiger and Kewallis, found the net for nine counters each, while Pelletier, in addition to holding his opposing forward scoreless, shot eight baskets. The French players were helpless and seldom had the ball. An entirely new American team was substituted in the last five minutes. Players follow: United States—Ruddiger (R.F.), Kewallis (L.F.), Brennan (C.), Pelletier (R.F.), Friedman (L.G.); substitutes, Greene, Clarke, May, Brown, and Doing. France—Bagay (R.F.), Aube (L.F.), Chauvet (C.), Turaglio (R.G.), Aguillaume (L.G.). (The Inter-Allied Games, The Games Committee, 1919)

Trying to Land on Both Feet

Zydrunas "Z" Ilgauskas

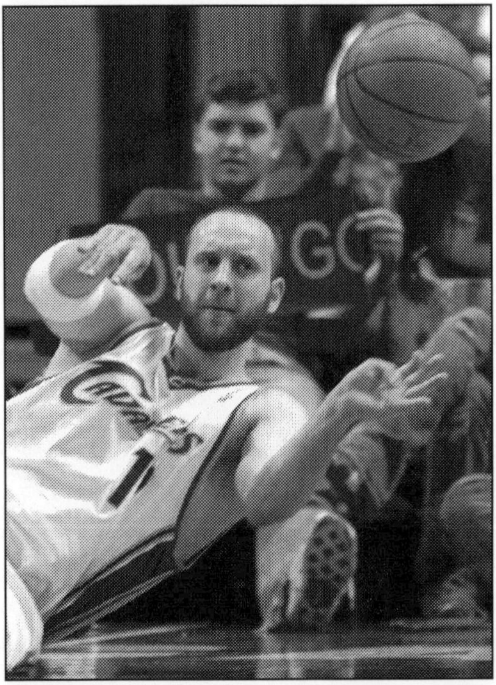

Born: 1975
Cleveland Cavaliers:
1997–2009
Position: Center
Jersey Number: 11

Zydrunas Ilgauskas passes to a teammate, 2006 (Courtesy *Akron Beacon Journal*)

SYMPTOMS

Zydrunas Ilgauskas played for the Lithuanian National Basketball team in the 1994 European Championships when he was twenty years old. He averaged a little over 7 points and rebounds per game. Standing seven foot three inches tall, Ilgauskas, known simply as "Z," idolized Arvydas Sabonis, the Lithuanian center who helped the Soviets beat the USA in the 1988 Olympics. Ilgauskas averaged 20.3 points, 12.8 rebounds, and 2.8 blocked shots playing for Atletas (Lithuanian League) during the 1995 season. However, he broke a bone in his foot and had to sit out the next year.

The Cavaliers still drafted him with their second first-round pick in the 1996 NBA draft and signed him to a reported three-year, $2.26-million deal. The following year he started 81 games and seemed to have put the injuries behind him. Ilgauskas inked a six-year, $70.87-million deal before the lockout-shortened 1998–99 season. Unfortunately, Z would only play in five games during the 1998 and 1999 seasons; during a February 1999 game against San Antonio, Ilgauskas broke a bone in his other foot (left foot).

In 2002, after slowly recovering from reconstructive surgeries, Z had his best season since joining the Cavs. He made the All-Star team while averaging 17.2 points and 7.5 rebounds per game. During LeBron James's 2004–05 rookie season, Ilgauskas was again chosen as an All-Star. The Cavs made the NBA Finals in 2007, but Ilgauskas did not have one of his better series, shooting only 35 percent from the floor as San Antonio easily triumphed. Since LeBron James was only in his third year, Cleveland fans were optimistic about a NBA Championship in the near future.

Ilgauskas continued to be a key contributor during the following seasons, but the team never got back to the finals. Before retiring, Z played a year with James in Miami, but a foot infection limited his playing time with the Heat. The Cavaliers retired his jersey in 2013 after a career where he averaged 13.8 points, 7.7 rebounds, and 1.6 blocks in 771 games. Big Z was a hardworking professional, something the area fans admired.

PATIENT HISTORY

"He can shoot. He can pass. He can rebound. It's a shame he lost so much time and so many games to these injuries. But we're going to see him blossom into something really, really good."
—Mike Fratello, Cavs coach

"Sometimes I think about what might have been if I hadn't been injured. I probably would have been a lot better player. I lost three or four years of my career."
—Zydrunas Ilgauskas

"He's been through so much. And it's nice to see him when he's happy. He loves the game of basketball, and it would mean so much to help him win a championship. He means a lot to me as a person."
—LeBron James

DIAGNOSIS

Ilgauskas became a fan favorite during his time in Cleveland. The Cavaliers stuck by him when he missed almost three of the first four years after signing a very large contract. Despite his injuries, he rehabbed diligently and came back to be a productive NBA player. When he had an opportunity to leave through free agency in 2005, he stuck by the Cavaliers, signing a five-year, $55-million contract extension to play with the team through the James era. Most fans remember the heartfelt embrace between Z and James after the Cavaliers finished off the Pistons in 2007.

Near the end of his career, Z was limited by his lack of foot speed and quickness. Multiple foot surgeries reduced his athleticism. Nevertheless, Ilgauskas did everything he could to help the team raise a championship banner in Cleveland, but in his fifteen years with the Cavaliers he could only raise the fans' hopes.

SECOND OPINION

Ilgauskas played in the postseason with the Cavaliers six times. In 71 games, he averaged a little over 28 minutes per contest and 11.0 points per outing. In the 2007 NBA Finals, Z averaged 7.8 points and 10.3 rebounds per game. Tim Duncan, the Spurs star center, posted better numbers—18.3 points and 11.5 rebounds per contest. Shooting at 44.4 percent, as compared to the Cavaliers 39.5 percent, the Spurs had little trouble sweeping the series and being crowned NBA Champions.

The series pointed out that the Cavaliers needed another consistent scorer. Unfortunately, due to trades in previous years, the Cavaliers did not have a 2007 draft pick. The following draft brought J. J. Hickson, a strong rebounder, to the team with the nineteenth pick. The outside threat the Cavaliers needed never materialized.

TREATMENT

Most stress fractures, or overload or fatigue fractures, heal with rest and rehabilitation. However, some are particularly problematic. One of the more difficult stress fractures to treat occurs in the tarsal navicular, a bone at the top of the midfoot. The injury was first described in the early 1970s and thought to be rare. However, due to advances in imaging, the fracture has become more widely reported.

The exact injury process is not known, though the injury is attributed to the fact that the navicular bone gets pinched or impinged between the bones to the front and back of it, causing it to be compressed. An athlete who has suffered a stress fracture at the top of the midfoot usually experiences the gradual onset of pain during athletic activities. Without treatment, the pain becomes progressively worse and occurs more frequently. Athletes often continue to play by altering their gait to take pressure off the midfoot.

X-rays often contribute to the confusion or delay in diagnosis, since the results are initially negative in about 60–70 percent of cases. The microfracture only shows up later, when the bone's healing response is detected. Advanced imaging, such as a bone scan or MRI, is necessary for a definitive diagnosis. CT scans show the best detail for this type of fracture. Because of the vague symptom presentation and confusing radiographic work up, an accurate diagnosis can take up to four months. The tarsal navicular is also an area of poor blood flow, making the bone susceptible to nonunion (nonhealing).

Early diagnosis makes treatment much easier. Resting in a non-weight-bearing cast is initially recommended. If the fracture fails to heal, surgery is necessary for athletes. A screw is normally used to fix midfoot fractures, but occasionally a bone graft is called for. Many athletes who combine running and jumping (football, basketball, track, etc.) are at high risk for stress fractures. Tall basketball players with large feet seem to have a particular propensity for these types of fractures.

INCIDENTAL FINDINGS

Among players from Lithuania who have played over 300 games in the NBA, Z leads the group with 843 games. Darius Songaila, a six foot nine center/power forward, played 495 games, primarily for Sacramento and Washington. At thirty one years old, the global star Arvydas Sabonis (470 games) signed with Portland and became Rookie of the Year. Linas "the Menace" Kleiza (409 games), a 2005 first-round draft pick, played for the Nuggets and Raptors. Sarunas Marciulionis (363 games), a shooting guard, had a seven-year NBA career, primarily with Golden State.

Above the Rim and Overweight

Shawn Kemp

Born: 1969
Cleveland Cavaliers: 1998–2000
Position: Power Forward / Center
Jersey Number: 4

SYMPTOMS

Basketball in Indiana is religion and Shawn Kemp was one of its many disciples at Concord High in Elkhart, Indiana, during the late 1980s. Rumors surfaced that the six-foot-eleven ninth-grader had once dunked over an Indiana Pacer who visited the school. People came to Concord's practices to see the high-flying prep star.

Bobby Knight wanted Kemp to go to Indiana University, but Kemp instead chose the University of Kentucky. For Hoosiers, this was sacrilege. Kemp never played at Kentucky, because he was academically ineligible and left the school after an incident at a local pawnshop. He transferred to Trinity Valley Community College in Athens, Texas, but only practiced with the team. After one year at two colleges, Kemp felt he was ready to play in the NBA.

In 1989, the Seattle Supersonics chose Kemp in the first round (seventeenth pick). He spent eight seasons with the Supersonics, averaging 16.2 points per game and 9.6 rebounds per game, and was an All-Star four times. During the 1995–96 season, Kemp's Supersonics lost to the Chicago Bulls in the NBA Finals. Due to his thunderous dunks, Kemp got the nickname "Reign Man" while playing in Seattle.

Eventually, Kemp wanted more money and asked to be traded. In a three-team swap prior to the 1997–98 season, Kemp and Sherman Douglas (Milwaukee Bucks) were sent to Cleveland. Cleveland shipped their All-Star point guard Terrel Brandon, Tyronne Hill, and their 1998 first-round draft pick to the Bucks. The Bucks traded Vin Baker to the Supersonics. Kemp signed a seven-year, $98-million contract with the Cavs.

Kemp's first season with the Cavaliers gave fans hope that the big man could become a cornerstone for a championship run. He led the team to the playoffs, and although the team lost in the first round to the Indiana Pacers, Kemp averaged 26 points and over 10 rebounds in the four-game affair. With a little help, the following season might prove even better.

Unfortunately, the owners locked out the players prior the 1998–99 season. After the labor dispute was settled, the league decided to go forward with a fifty-game schedule. Kemp reported to training camp severely overweight; according to reports, the Cavalier had gained at least thirty-four pounds if not closer to sixty. Kemp still managed to score over 20 points a game, but the team finished at 22–28 and out of the playoffs. Fans and management alike wondered what they were getting for Kemp's big contract. After the season, Mike Fratello was fired and Wayne Embry, who had been named the *Sporting News* NBA Executive of the Year the previous season, was forced to step down.

In August 2000, Cleveland unloaded Kemp and his large contract and Portland became his new NBA home. In a three-way deal that also involved the Miami Heat, Portland sent Brian Grant to Miami and Cleveland-native Gary Grant to the Cavs. Miami sent Chris Gatling and Clarence Weatherspoon to Cleveland, along with a first-round draft choice and cash. The Cavs used the pick to select Brendan Haywood and traded his signing rights to the Orlando Magic for Michael Doleac, who played one season with Cleveland.

Kemp never regained his All-Star form and was soon out of the NBA. Cleveland faced several miserable seasons and a round robin of coaches. However, the Cavaliers bad play eventually led to the lottery pick and LeBron James.

PATIENT HISTORY

"Teams that got to the top in this league invariably did a deal out of the ordinary. The Celtics got Bird that way [by selecting him as a junior-eligible, a year before he came out]. And we think getting Shawn can be that kind of deal for us."
—Bob Whitsitt, Seattle Supersonics general manager

"He was really very honest about it [weight gain]. I said, 'Shawn, how did this happen?' He said, 'Coach, I didn't think we were coming back.'"
—Mike Fratello, Cavs coach

"When I dunk, I just want to tear the rim down."
—Shawn Kemp

DIAGNOSIS

After the great Cavaliers teams of the late the 1980s and early 1990s were dismantled, every fan knew it would take time for the team to rebuild. In 1993, the Cavaliers hired Mike Fratello to put the pieces together. Fratello preached a team game and strong defense. Hoping to speed up the restructuring, the Cavs traded for Shawn Kemp, a twenty-eight-year-old, six-time All-Star. Kemp, unfortunately, chewed and swallowed more than he should have. While Kemp's weight went higher, the team's play dropped lower. Kemp's lack of success also delivered a severe blow to Mike Fratello's coaching career and the Cavaliers' fortunes. This led to the team becoming an annual attendee at the NBA draft lottery.

SECOND OPINION

Perhaps if Wayne Embry had gotten his wish, Shawn Kemp might not have ended up in a Cleveland uniform. Kemp was not the Cavs general manager's first choice. The team couldn't keep either Chris Mills or Bobby Phills in the fold. Offers to Boston's Rick Fox and Sacramento's Brian Grant were snubbed; both players went elsewhere for a little less money.

Another issue was attendance. Attendance had dropped from eleventh in the league in 1995–96 to sixteenth in the league in 1996–97. Without some additional fire power on offense (the team had finished last in points scored in the season prior to Kemp's arrival) prospects for a packed Gund Arena didn't look promising.

Kemp's salary was a big price to pay for one playoff season. As Kemp grew in girth, he was less of a factor on the court. He also became a burden off the court—arriving late for games, team meetings, and flights. Perhaps these were early signs of his personality issues and addiction problems.

TREATMENT

Obesity is a difficult, complex, and multifaceted medical condition; it is not easily treated or cured. Nearly one-third of Americans are overweight or obese. The health consequences of obesity include increased risk of heart disease, high blood pressure, stroke, arthritis, certain cancers, sleep apnea, and depression. Obesity decreases life expectancy by six to seven years. It is particularly difficult for athletes and is frequently associated with a rapid decline in performance.

The body mass index is used to determine an individual's classification on a scale of underweight to severely overweight. The two measurements that are needed are height in inches and weight in pounds. The formula to calculate BMI is

$$(\text{weight}/\text{height}^2) \times 703$$

For example, a male who stands six feet tall (72 inches) and weighs 210 pounds would have a BMI of 28.47.

$$(210 / (72 \times 72)) \times 703 = 28.47$$

Table 1. BMI classifications according to the World Health Organization

Classification	BMI
Underweight	Less than 18.5
Normal Weight	18.5—24.99
Overweight	25—29.99
Obesity (Class I)	30—34.99
Obesity (Class II)	35—39.99
Obesity (Class III)	40.0 or greater

Among the treatments for obesity are lifestyle modification (including dietary and physical activity and exercise) and behavioral therapy (including goal setting, self-monitoring, stimulus control, problem solving, relapse control, and cognitive restructuring). Better results are attained "through a combination of strategies that target dietary therapy, exercise and physical activity, and use of group sessions for behavioral therapy" (*Journal of Nursing Scholarship* 43, no. 4, (2011): 368–75). Other options include pharmacotherapy and bariatric surgery procedures like gastric bypass and gastric banding.

INCIDENTAL FINDINGS

Recommendations on food intake in relationship to sports have a long history. For example, in the early 1920s, advice was not lacking.

> When it comes to actual figures to express the needs of the body for severe muscular work, we can, of course, only deal with averages. . . . The following figures are presented so that there may be compared to some diets actually in use with standards expressive of the body's requirement during severe muscular exercise.

Activity	Protein	Fat	Carbohydrate	Calories
Rowing average of six crews	155 gm. (5 oz.)	177 gm. (6 oz.)	440 gm. (14½ oz.)	4085
Football average of two teams	225 gm. (7½ oz.)	354 gm. (12 oz.)	633 gm. (21 oz.)	6812
Standard (Voit*) hard muscular work	145 gm. (5 oz.)	100 gm. (3½ oz.)	450 gm. (15 oz.)	3370
Hard muscular work (Playfair**)	185 gm. (6 oz.)	71 gm. (21/3 oz.)	568 gm. (19 oz.)	3750

* Developed by Carl Voit of Germany.
** Developed by Lyon Playfair of England.
(Material adapted from *Nutrition and Clinical Dietetics*, 2nd ed., Philadelphia: Lea & Febiger, 1921.)

Bringing It All Home

LeBron Raymone "King" or "Chosen One" James

Born: 1984
Cleveland Cavaliers: 2003–09
Position: Small Forward / Guard
Jersey Number: 23

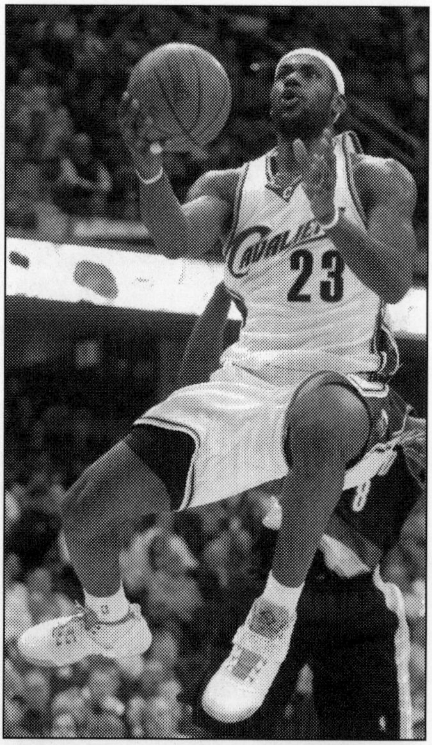

LeBron James scoops to the hoop, 2008 (Courtesy *Akron Beacon Journal*)

SYMPTOMS

Upon entering Akron, Ohio, from any number of directions, a sign will let you know that the former "Rubber Capital of the World" is the hometown of the LeBron James. James now has a house in Bath, one of Akron's tony suburbs, but his heart remains with Akron, where he grew up as the son of a single mom. Recently he donated $1 million for a gym at his high school alma mater. He hosts an annual bikeathon to raise money for charity, and supports the Akron public schools with funding for educational programs and technology needs. While James's charity is unquestioned, some fans in

Northeast Ohio are ambivalent toward the star, and some even feel he left them as cold as a stiff winter wind blowing in off of Lake Erie after he moved to warm Miami. His recent return has brought renewed hope, and resilient Cleveland fans are waiting to celebrate an NBA Championship.

James started getting press locally as a six-foot-four freshman at St. Vincent-St. Mary High School (the Fighting Irish). He led his team in scoring (17.7 points a game), rebounds (5.92), assists (3.56), steals (3.16), and blocked shots (22). The undefeated Irish won the 2002 Division III State Championship and were ranked twenty-first nationally. The following year, James became nationally prominent by being the first high school sophomore to be named to the *USA Today* All-USA First Team, leading his team to a second state championship. He continued his stellar career at St. Vincent-St. Mary, winning another state championship as a senior while averaging 31.6 points, 9.6 rebounds, 4.6 assists, and 3.4 steals per game. James was physically gifted; he chose to forego college and enter the 2003 NBA draft.

The Cavaliers dismal 2002–03 season put them in the lottery for the number one overall pick. Tied with Denver for the best odds (225 chances out of 1000) to garner the pick, Cleveland's fortunes seemed to change dramatically when they won the LeBron James lottery. Not since Bernie Kosar, another Ohio kid who came home to play for the Browns, was the fans' fervor so palpable. With James in the Cavaliers lineup, undoubtedly an NBA Championship might finally become a reality.

After missing the playoffs in James's rookie and second seasons, the Cavaliers became postseason perennials, but the expected championship never materialized. Even with the NBA's best regular season record several times, the team made the NBA Finals only once, in 2007, and lost to the San Antonio Spurs in four games. In one final effort to move Cleveland to the Promised Land, the Cavaliers acquired Shaquille O'Neal during King James's final year before he was eligible for free agency. During the 2009–10 season, the Cavaliers finished with the league's best record, 61–21. In the first round of the playoffs, the Cavs easily got by the Chicago Bulls.

In the next series, the Cavaliers faced the Celtics, the team that had eliminated them from the postseason in 2008. After winning game one, the Cavaliers lost the second game and home court advantage. James had a poor game and seemed lethargic at times. He was suffering from a strained and bruised right elbow, an injury that seemed to be affecting his outside shot. In game three, James rebounded with 38 points and the Cavs took a 2–1 series lead.

James's on again-off again series was off in a game four loss in Boston. Game five was even worse, as James only managed 15 points on 3-of-14 shooting. The final act in the first LeBron James era was a tragedy; Cleveland lost game six. James's stat line for the final game included 27 points, a career-playoff-high 19 rebounds, and 10 assists, but King James only shot 8 out of 21 from the floor and turned the ball over 9 times. Rumors about bickering on the team and with the coaching staff surfaced after the Celtics' victory.

In the off-season, Cleveland fans were shocked again. James chose to leave the area and sign with the Miami Heat. With Chris Bosh and Dwayne Wade, James secured his dream of being an NBA Champion. Even as a Heat player, James spent a large amount of time and money on local charitable activities, including his "Wheels for Education" program.

PATIENT HISTORY

> "He's one of the best freshmen you'll ever see."
> —Keith Dambrot, James's high school coach

> "There's no question in Game 5 [2010 playoff series against Boston] LeBron was kind of out of it. I always believed he could turn it on at any moment, but for some reason he didn't."
> —Shaquille O'Neal

"I don't really put a title on it [charitable giving]. I do it because I have a passion. I do it because I want to do it. It's not because someone came to me and said, 'You should do this because you owe it to them.' It's something that was instilled in me to give back. This is my city [Akron, Ohio], there's 190,000 of us. For me to be one of the few to make it, it wasn't hard at all."
—LeBron James

DIAGNOSIS

The youngest of the Cleveland major sports teams, the Cavaliers have experienced some incredible highs ("Miracle of Richfield") and some incredible lows (from 1999 through 2002, the team had a record of 108 wins against 220 losses). The ultimate prize of the dismal run was winning the lottery pick that landed LeBron James.

When the Cavaliers drafted James in 2003, Cleveland fans were convinced that James would lead Cleveland to one, if not many, NBA Championships. An Akron native, area fans had been well aware of the super talent LeBron possessed. When that talent didn't produce NBA Championships immediately, diehard fans pointed out that it took seven years for Michael Jordan to win his first NBA Championship with the Chicago Bulls. The first LeBron era failed to bring Cleveland a title, but it did bring a level of excitement and media attention that hadn't been seen in Northeast Ohio for decades.

Fans wondered what could have been if Carlos Boozer had stayed with the team instead of "tricking" team owners into letting him out of his contract early. Boozer's departure meant LeBron never played with a secondary star, a formula that could have helped the team get to the top of the NBA. After Boozer left, the team went through a merry-go-round of perimeter shooters who seemed to lose their three-point touch in Cleveland, including Damon Jones, Donyell Marshall, and Wally Szczerbiak.

Management tried to help LeBron by securing some big men. However, Zydrunas Ilgauskas' body and skills were deteriorating and the additions of Ben Wallace and Shaquille O'Neal did not help the team as much as expected. In hindsight, if Cleveland had had Shaq prior to the 2009 Eastern Conference Finals versus Orlando, Dwight Howard might not have averaged almost 26 points and 13 rebounds in the series, including 40 points in the sixth game. In James's first era with Cleveland, getting Amaré Stoudemire instead of Antawn Jamison at the trade deadline might have pushed the team past Boston and toward an NBA Championship.

For many fans, the greatest mystery of the first LeBron Era is how the 2010 Eastern Conference Semifinal against Boston ended in defeat. All fans love conspiracy theories, and many reasons were given to explain LeBron's performance, but undoubtedly his elbow injury, suffered in the earlier series against Chicago, played a role in the final outcome. NBA experts did point out that the Celtics defense was equipped to put James and the rest of the Cavaliers offense in a stranglehold. The Big Three (Paul Pierce, Kevin Garnett, and Ray Allen), along with Kendrick Perkins and Rajon Rondo, executed Tom Thibodeau's brilliant defensive strategy, playing a quasi-zone against the Cavaliers to shut down the Cavaliers' offensive advantage. During Thibodeau's tenure in Boston, James averaged 26.7 points, but shot just 39.4 percent from the field and 24.6 percent from the three-point line in 13 postseason games. LeBron might not have been at 100 percent, but the Celtics' defense was.

Coaching was not considered to be a distinct advantage for the Cavaliers, despite the team's strong regular season records. Although Mike Brown brought defense and toughness to the franchise, he was overmatched in bench coaching, game strategy, and offensive game plans. In the 2009 playoffs, Stan Van Gundy of the Orlando Magic severely outcoached Brown during the conference finals. After the series loss, Cavaliers management considered replacing Brown, who had been selected as the NBA Coach of the Year. The team kept Brown in place, but unfortunately, in the 2010 playoffs Brown was out-coached by Doc Rivers, allowing the Boston Celtics to beat the favored Cavaliers.

LeBron's elbow problem dated back to April, causing him to miss the team's final four regular season games. General Manager Danny Ferry said the elbow injury was severe enough during the playoffs that, had it been a regular season game, the team would have sat out the Cleveland star. James was eventually diagnosed with a sprain and a bone bruise. The injury limited James's ability to handle the basketball. He tried several braces and pads without much success. James received daily treatments, including electric stimulation, heat, ice, and various forms of physical therapy.

James was frank about his injury, saying that he would soldier on. He was, however, concerned because he indicated that he didn't actually know what the injury was. James described the problem as if someone hit his funny bone and the elbow numbed up. X-rays and an MRI showed no obvious structural damage. Some Cleveland fans didn't buy the explanation; in their view, James knew he was going to leave via free agency and faked the injury.

James clearly played differently in the Boston series than for most of his other 600 games as a Cavalier. He did not handle the ball, drive the ball, or dunk with his right hand; his shooting, particularly from long range, was flat without much backspin. James's rebound and assist totals were indicative of his career numbers, but his scoring and shooting percentage dropped significantly. He shot over 50 percent in the playoffs in 2008 and 2009, but shot only 45 percent during the Boston series. James shot only 27 percent from three-point range during the Boston series, a drop from his typical 33 percent.

A couple months later, James compounded Cleveland's playoff loss pain by making "The Decision." The nationally televised event was vilified by fans from all parts of the country and sports writers, and James's public image took a significant hit.

After proclaiming that he would bring a championship to Cleveland, James had captured the hearts of most Cleveland fans. They celebrated his roots when he held his NBA Most Valuable Player ceremonies in Akron at St. Vincent-St. Mary High School and The University of Akron. Fans were happy that these places meant something to their NBA superstar. James's dreams were Cleveland's dreams.

Obviously, the Cleveland fan base was devastated when James gave up on his chase for a Cleveland championship and left for greener pastures. Michael Jordan and Magic Johnson hadn't run away to make their dreams come true. Most fans felt James didn't have the intestinal fortitude to finish the job of winning in Cleveland, and the blatant formation of a Miami "Dream Team" was a way to fabricate a championship.

Cleveland fans, used to situations like the Browns departure to Baltimore, bounced back resiliently. The local sports media began to discuss the best players available in the upcoming NBA Draft. One small moment of revenge did come the following season when the Cavaliers handed the Heat a 102–90 loss late in the 2010–11 season. The area fans were also jubilant when their adopted team, the Dallas Mavericks, beat the Heat in that year's NBA Finals. The ability to withstand the crushing blows of the summer of 2010 only strengthened the resolve and enduring hope of the Cleveland fans.

SECOND OPINION

The issues surrounding LeBron James and taking his "talents to South Beach" will never be resolved to Cavaliers' fans liking. However, some blame has to be attributed to the team's management for the ultimate departure of the "King." James never had a secondary star (Shaq was at the end of his career when he came to Cleveland) who could pick up the offensive slack so opposing teams, especially in the playoffs, couldn't double- and triple-team James.

Comparing James to players like Magic Johnson or Kobe Bryant—who stayed with one team their entire careers—is not quite fair. By the time Johnson was in his third year as a Laker, the team had won two NBA crowns. Kobe Bryant, after the Lakers brought in Phil Jackson, a proven winner, lifted the NBA Championship trophy in his fourth year. Michael Jordan, who played for the Bulls almost his entire career, might be most similar to James, but even those comparisons aren't really applicable. Jordan sat out most of his second year with a broken foot, setting the star back a season. In his third year, the Bulls hired Doug Collins, who had played in the NBA as a shooting guard, to develop Jordan. In Jordan's sixth season, Collins was replaced by Phil Jackson, and the Bulls, with Scottie Pippen in the lineup, began to win NBA titles shortly thereafter.

Cavs' ownership never pulled the plug on Mike Brown, even though he was out-coached on several occasions in the playoffs. Brown's short tenure with the Lakers tells volumes about his ability to deal with superstars. His recent one-year return to Cleveland didn't work out well either.

Good or bad, LeBron James will be judged on how many championships he wins during his career. Fans in Cleveland wouldn't have been thrilled if he stayed and the team continued to be ousted before winning it all. LeBron remains loyal to his hometown and he surely is trying to prove that "You Can Go Home Again" since he has recently rejoined the team. Will he be able to lead the Cavaliers to an NBA crown?

TREATMENT

Elbow injuries (see medical illustrations, pages 303–304) occur frequently in all sports. Traumatic injuries such as fractures or ligament tears are usually acute and easily diagnosed by using X-rays or advanced imaging techniques like MRIs. Overuse injuries (overload or stress) usually last a few weeks, unless they are chronic. These injuries may not always be as readily apparent or as easy to diagnose.

There are four common types of sports-related elbow injuries that do not exhibit structured ligament tears or fractures: medial epicondylitis; ulnar nerve entrapment or compression syndrome; deep bruising with olecranon bursitis, elbow contusion, and bone bruise; and ulnar collateral ligament (UCL) sprain.

Medial epicondylitis (sometimes referred to as golfer's elbow) is an overload injury to the tendon and bony attachment on the inside of the elbow, which occurs on the opposite side of the area associated with the more common "tennis elbow." The injury is caused by a series of microtears of the tendon caused by repetitive work or sports-related activities, such as a golf swing, baseball pitch, or shooting a basketball. An X-ray may rule out arthritis or bone chips but not show a tendon injury. Even an MRI may not provide specific findings. After weeks or months of overuse, the tendon can develop scar tissue with decreased blood flow or tendonosis (damage to the inner layers of a tendon on the cellular level). Weakness or poor endurance develops in high demand activities. Tendon rupture can be the worst complication.

Treatment includes rest or eliminating the activities that caused the problem. When athletes continue to play through the injury, anti-inflammatory medicines may help; an elbow strap or brace may be helpful as well. Physical therapy includes deep tissue massage (to break up scar tissue), ultrasound treatments (to reduce pain and swelling), and muscle stimulation (to reduce overload trauma until resting). Cortisone injections (steroids) are a last resort to reduce swelling or promote healing. Steroids can weaken the tendon, however, so injections must be used with caution.

The newest injection technique, known as PRP (platelet rich plasma), is supposed to stimulate new tissue growth. PRP is gaining widespread popularity, especially in college and professional athletes. Studies on long-term results have not yet been extensively conducted.

The ulnar nerve injury in the elbow (ulnar nerve entrapment or compression syndrome) is second only to carpal tunnel syndrome as a source of nerve pain in the arm. The nerve, located around the back and inside of the elbow, can be stretched, bruised, pinched (entrapped), inflamed (ulnar neuritis), or slip out of place (sublux). Early symptoms of ulnar nerve injuries include aching pain, numbness, and tingling in the ring and little fingers. Later, weakness develops, which can cause hand clumsiness or cramping and hinder opening a jar, turning a key, or playing sports.

The diagnosis for ulnar nerve injures depend largely on a physical exam. The results of the exam may not always show the presence of an injury. X-rays are helpful only if bone chips or bone spurs are present from recurrent trauma. In most cases, X-rays and advanced imaging techniques do not show specific results. EMG/NCT (electromyography/nerve conduction) tests may show nerve injuries or reductions in nerve velocity in persistent cases. However, many sports-related nerve injuries are dynamic (i.e., they only occur with certain movements) and, therefore, even NCTs show normal results.

Treatment for this injury involves modifying a patient's activities or resting. An elbow splint worn at night or a brace worn during activity can help protect the elbow and the nerve. Anti-inflammatory medicines may help, but cortisone injections are not recommended. Surgical decompression (exploring the nerve in the region of the elbow and removing any forces that "push on" it) of the nerve is indicated for advanced cases or when rest and bracing alone do not relieve pressure.

Trauma from a blow or recurrent hits on the elbow can cause bruising to the soft tissues, the bone, or the bursal sac, known as deep bruising with olecranon bursitis, elbow contusion, and bone bruise. This bruising, especially to the bursal sac, can cause significant swelling, with a large blood collection that reduces range of motion of the elbow. The broken blood vessels take time to heal and repeated trauma can prevent the injury from healing correctly. Infection is another complication of recurrent contusions.

Treatment includes rest and preventing further trauma to the elbow. If significant blood is in the bursal sac, aspiration (drainage) with a needle can speed up the healing process and allow an athlete to continue to play. An injection may also speed relief for an athlete. A bone bruise usually takes a longer period (several months) of rest to heal. A brace or protective pad can also assist in the treatment phase.

A sprain (tear) of the ulnar collateral ligament (UCL) in the elbow is frequently discussed in sports medicine. Although a tear of this ligament may happen with a "pop" and a single episode of trauma, a gradual onset of pain on the inside of the elbow is more common. With a gradual injury, there is an initial partial tear and stretch injury to the triangular ligament that supports the inside of the elbow. Although this occurs most frequently in throwing sports like baseball, the ligament sprain can also occur in contact sports such as wrestling, football, and basketball.

The diagnosis of UCL injuries is still somewhat complex. The physical exam may show swelling and bruising within the area of the ligament, but this depends on the timing of the injury and whether the injury is acute or chronic. Stress tests may show looseness or laxity in the elbow; elbow looseness, however, is difficult to determine clinically. X-rays are useful mainly in ruling out problems, such as bone chips, in the joint that can mimic torn ligaments.

Treatment is very similar to that of an MCL tear in the knee or an ankle sprain. Initial rest and bracing, followed by aggressive strengthening exercises in physical therapy, help athletes return to play sooner. The athlete may not return at 100 percent capability and may require a brace or taping to help support the healing ligaments. The treatment for throwing athletes is different, because of the stress demand placed on the inside of the elbow under maximum effort pitches. A reconstructive surgery of this ligament (Tommy John surgery, see page 108) may be recommended for young pitchers and some field position players (especially catchers) who cannot return to throwing at maximum velocity with physical therapy alone. Most athletes manage without the need for surgery.

INCIDENTAL FINDINGS

Tennis became very popular in the late 1800s, due to the fact that Charles Goodyear invented a process for rubber called vulcanization. The process allowed tennis balls to bounce higher and the game was able to be played outdoors on grass. As muscles in the arm became overused, a new malady arose—lawn tennis arm:

> Mr. Henry Morris (*Lancet*, July 29, 1882) describes a sprain of the pronator radii teres muscle [located on the palm side of the

> forearm] due to playing lawn tennis. This sprain, Mr. Morris believes, is the result of the frequent back stroke whereby the forearm is brought into rapid and forcible pronation. The condition is slight swelling, with tenderness on firm pressure along the course of the pronator and pain in bringing the muscle into action, but, as a rule, not otherwise. If the forearm is enveloped in an elastic bandage or firm elastic webbing, and kept at rest, the symptoms soon disappear. (*Canadian Medical Journal* 11 (1883): 95)

Typically, new remedies also came about:

> For this affection [lawn tennis arm] a correspondent of the *Lancet* recommends chaulmoogra [an Asian tree] oil carefully rubbed into the arm at night and morning. This oil, he states, is now generally used by men after their first day's hunting, and also by bicyclists after their first day's long ride, because they find that it entirely prevents any irritation of the skin or stiffness if it is well rubbed in before they retire to bed. (*Med. Record*, Sept. 23)

An Up and Down Career

Delonte Maurice West

Born: 1983
Cleveland Cavaliers: 2007–09
Position: Guard
Jersey Number: 13

SYMPTOMS

Delonte West's childhood was one of constant relocation. His mother and his siblings moved from place to place and stayed with anyone who could put them up. West went to at least four different elementary and middle schools in the Washington, DC area. Even though he didn't play organized basketball, shooting hoops was a calming constant in his life. West developed a deft touch and might have remained in the shadows except for a chance incident. While shooting hoops outside of Eleanor Roosevelt High School in Maryland, members of the basketball team pointed West out to the coach, who asked West to show up to practice the next day. He did and became a starter for the team.

West wasn't recruited heavily by any Division 1 schools. He eventually took an offer from St. Joseph's University in Philadelphia and majored in art. On the court, West was paired with Jameer Nelson, whose name is plastered all over the St. Joseph's record books. In 2004, senior Nelson and junior West made up arguably the best back court in college basketball at a school with an enrollment of less than 5,000 students. West averaged 18.9 points and 6.7 assists per game and shot 41 percent from three-point range. The Hawks started the season at 27–0 and were ranked number one in the country. In the NCAA basketball tournament, St. Joseph's made it to the Elite Eight before losing a two-point decision to Oklahoma State. West led all scorers in the game, pouring in 20 points.

Foregoing his senior year, West was drafted twenty-fourth overall by the Boston Celtics. After a short career in Boston, West was dealt to the Seattle Supersonics, with Wally Szczerbiak and the rights to Jeff Green, for Ray Allen. In 2008, West became a Cavalier as part of a three-way trade between the Cavs, the Bulls, and the Supersonics. The Cavaliers were looking to bolster their lineup for a playoff run. West averaged over 10 points a game as the Cavs defeated the Washington Wizards in the first round of the playoffs and over 11 points a game against Boston in the Eastern Conference Semifinals, but the Cavs ultimately lost.

The following season, the LeBron James-led Cavaliers scorched the league during the regular season, compiling a 66–16 record. Delonte West became a permanent fixture at the starting shooting guard position. During the playoffs, West upped his contribution, averaging 15 points a game in series against the Atlanta Hawks and Orlando Magic. The team, however, couldn't get by Dwight Howard and the hot three-point shooting Magics. Fans were disappointed, but were excited about the future.

Unfortunately, West's career began to unravel during the off-season. In September 2009, he was stopped in Maryland and was found to be carrying three guns—a Beretta 9mm in West's waistband, a Ruger .357 magnum strapped to his leg, and a shotgun in a guitar case slung over his back. West eventually plead guilty to two weapons counts and avoided jail; he was sentenced to eight months home detention, two-months' probation, and forty hours community service. The weight of the Maryland incident was exacerbated by the realization that West was battling bipolar disorder and might not have been on his medications during the police stop.

The Cavaliers treated West's condition, but his play became inconsistent and at times he was placed on the inactive list. His scoring production also dropped. The final blow was an unsubstantiated rumor that West was having a relationship with Gloria James, LeBron's mother. The team's chemistry fell apart in the Eastern Conference Semifinal loss against Boston. Before the 2010–11 season, West was traded, along with guard Sebastian Telfair, to the Minnesota Timberwolves for point guard Ramon Sessions, Ryan Hollins, and a future second-round pick.

PATIENT HISTORY

> "The real message is that this is a young man [West] who has stepped forward and been able to say that, 'I have been diagnosed with this [bipolar disorder].' And on top of that, he is making a concerted effort to doing what needs to be done to have a good outcome."
> —Dr. Thomas Eppright

> "Oh, man. Playing in the Q. The best arena in the league. When I left Cleveland and went to other places, guys would talk about how hard it was to play in Cleveland, and how fun it was. It was unbelievable. There was so much energy in the city."
> —Delonte West

> "Delonte thinks he is a smooth guy. Silky smooth. But that's his personality. Nice guy. Dresses nice. Always wearing ties and dress slacks."
> —Jameer Nelson, St. Joseph's teammate

DIAGNOSIS

The Cavaliers had the league's best record in 2008–09 and West's role was a key to the team's success. In 2009–10, West got off to a very slow start and missed some games, reportedly due to a bipolar disorder. His mental illness played a role in his off-court issues, and Cavs fans wondered if that disorder was impacting on-court chemistry. During the team's final season with James, the Cavaliers unraveled against the Celtics. Following the series loss, the team was dismantled in the wake of LeBron James's "Decision" to sign with the

Miami Heat. Without James in Cleveland, the Cavaliers finished with the second-worst record in the NBA in 2011 and ended up in the NBA draft lottery. Fans had to watch the team start over again.

SECOND OPINION

West's part in the Boston series loss should be viewed in context. If fingers need to be pointed, Antawn Jamison scored over 7 points less per game in the Boston series than he had during the Cavs' 4–1 series victory over the Chicago Bulls. LeBron James scored 5 points less per game, too. Many fans thought that Boston coach Doc Rivers did a better job preparing his team and designed a strategy that forced the other Cavaliers to beat the Celtics, instead of just James. The James's impending free agency, undoubtedly, placed undue stress on the team. The sad part is Delonte West could have been a reliable, steady player in the NBA.

TREATMENT

See discussion of bipolar disorder, page 32.

INCIDENTAL FINDINGS

Coleman Roberts Griffith (1893–1966) is considered the father of sports psychology in the United States. In 1938, P. K. Wrigley, the owner of the Chicago Cubs, had Griffith set up a laboratory to determine how best to identify the personal, muscular, and mental attributes that great athletes possess and how to identify the traits in potential ballplayers.

In reports produced for the Cubs owner, Griffith proposed creating achievement tests for measuring the speed, strength, coordination, accuracy, and visual judgment of players. He suggested using the tests to judge minor league talent and to track players' progress (or decline) and prescribe specific exercises to develop the skills most in need of improvement. In a rather interesting notion, one that baseball "men" of the time discounted, Griffith contended that committing errors damaged the confidence of the players involved, "subconsciously" affecting the player's performance, possibly for many days afterward.

Thumbs Up

Shaquille Rashaun "Shaq" "Diesel" "The Big Aristotle" "Big Cactus" O'Neal

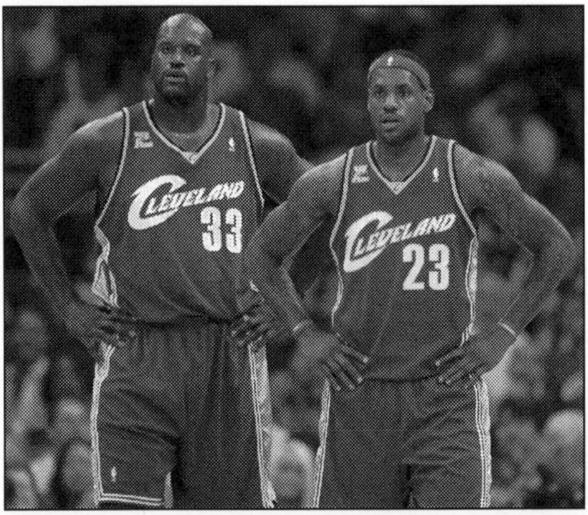

Born: 1972
Cleveland Cavaliers: 2009
Position: Center
Jersey Number: 33

LeBron James and Shaquille O'Neal on the floor together, 2009 (Courtesy *Akron Beacon Journal*)

SYMPTOMS

By the age of thirty-seven, Shaquille "Shaq" O'Neal had quite literally done it all in the NBA. He had been the Rookie of the Year, won four championship rings, won three consecutive finals MVP awards, was the league's Most Valuable Player in 2000, and was named to the NBA All-Star team fifteen times. He was called "Diesel," "The Big Aristotle," and "Big Cactus." And standing over seven foot tall and weighing 325 pounds, why not. In 2009, the Cavaliers hoped Shaq's broad shoulders, along with LeBron James's scoring prowess, would lead to a championship parade down Euclid Avenue.

At the age of fourteen, O'Neal was six foot eight. He was spotted by LSU coach Dale Brown, who was on a speaking tour in Germany (where O'Neal's stepfather was stationed). After moving to San Antonio, O'Neal starred at Cole High School. In his senior year, his team went 36–0 and won the 1989 Texas 3A Championship. O'Neal averaged over 32 points and 22 rebounds a game and was named a McDonald's and *Parade* magazine All-American.

The meeting with Brown prompted O'Neal to attend LSU, where he was a major force on the hardwood. Among his numerous accomplishments, he became the first player to lead the Southeastern Conference in scoring, rebounding, field goal percentage, and blocked shots in the same season, and he was chosen as the Associated Press National Player of the Year and the SEC Athlete of the Year in 1991. He became the first overall pick of the Orlando Magic in the 1992 NBA draft. O'Neal also won a gold medal in the 1996 Olympic Games in Atlanta.

In the summer of 2009, the Cavaliers acquired Shaq from the Phoenix Suns for Ben Wallace, Sasha Pavlovic, and cash. Early in the season, O'Neal missed several games with a shoulder injury. By the end of the season, the Cavaliers had finished with a 61–21 record, good enough for first place in the Central Division. However, O'Neal suffered a significant thumb injury in a February 25, 2010, game against Boston and was forced to sit out the rest of the season after undergoing surgery.

Shaq returned for the Cavaliers' playoff run. In the first round, the Cavaliers easily beat the Bulls, 4–1. Next up were the Boston Celtics. During the season, the Cavaliers had lost twice to the Celtics and won only once. A path to the conference final looked open when the Cavaliers took a 2–1 series lead, even though they lost game two and the home court advantage. Then the team collapsed, losing three straight games and chance at an NBA ring. O'Neal had subpar performances in games one and two, shooting a combined 8 for 22 and grabbing only 8 rebounds. In game three, he scored 12 points and pulled down 9 rebounds. He had 17 points in game four, 21 points in game five, but only 11 points in game six. He was not a presence on the boards in the final three games, averaging less than 5 rebounds per game.

The loss to Boston ended the first LeBron James era in Cleveland. The $20-million investment for Shaq didn't turn out as expected.

The Cavs had hoped to hitchhike a ride to an NBA crown, but Shaq's thumb injury sent them down a different highway.

PATIENT HISTORY

> "He is a force. He always has been. Still is. On the defensive end, just around the basket, he's a wall. Offensively he's a force in that he's going to get double teams."
> —Danny Ferry, Cavaliers general manager

> "He changed the game, just like Wilt Chamberlain did, by being so overpowering. Shaq was quick, strong, and unbelievably athletic. He was almost impossible to guard."
> —Alvin Gentry, Phoenix Suns coach

> "We got used to playing without Shaq, and it's great that we proved we can do that. But it's a little bit like when you're reading and you think the light's fine, and then somebody comes along and turns on a big, bright lamp. You say to yourself, 'Wow, that's much better, isn't it?'"
> —Horace Grant, Orlando power forward

DIAGNOSIS

The Cleveland Cavaliers found their back against the wall in the summer of 2009. LeBron James, Cleveland's superstar and reigning NBA Most Valuable Player, was in the final year of his contract. With free agency looming, the Cavaliers decided to go all out to win the NBA Championship. During the previous season, the Orlando Magic knocked out the Cavaliers in the conference semifinals, even after Cleveland compiled the best regular season record. Orlando center Dwight Howard overpowered the Cavaliers, and the team needed a big body to match up with him. Shaq, one of the all-time strongest NBA players, was clearly the man for the job. He came to Cleveland motivated to win a fifth championship ring. He quickly proclaimed that Cleveland no longer needed to double-team Howard. His motto was simple: "Win a ring for the King."

At times the strategy seemed to work, as the Cavaliers played much better during the regular season against the Los Angeles Lakers and the Orlando Magic. At other times, the team's chemistry appeared to be a major problem and the offense slowed down to the lumbering pace of the aging center. On February 25, 2010, O'Neal suffered a severe right thumb injury while attempting a shot against Boston Celtics center Glen "Big Baby" Davis. O'Neal had surgery on the thumb on March 1, and did not return until the first round of the playoffs against the Chicago Bulls. The Cavaliers struggled to find their rhythm with the big center in the game. On May 13, the Cavaliers were eliminated from the playoffs, losing to the Boston Celtics 4–2 in the Eastern Conference Semifinals. Injuries may have had an effect on his season, but Shaq averaged career lows in almost every major statistical category.

To use the word "implosion" would understate the Cavaliers' disaster in the 2010 playoffs. The role of Shaq's injury, presence in the lineup, and lack of production will be debated by Cleveland fans for decades. He spoke highly of his time in Cleveland and he endeared himself to most of the basketball fans in the city. No matter how admired Shaq was off the court, his year in Cleveland will go down as one of the most disappointing seasons in Cleveland sports history.

SECOND OPINION

Cleveland's loss to the Celtics can't be solely attributed to Shaq. The Cavaliers (50 total offensive rebounds/180 total defensive rebounds) matched Boston (56 total offensive rebounds/183 total defensive rebounds) on the boards. Boston shot better from the field (.470 to .450), and in several games Boston was superb from beyond the three-point arc. The Cavs couldn't match the Celtics' three-point output.

The real problem for the 2010 Cavs was that they turned the ball over 17 more times in the series than the Celtics and the Celtics had 43 more field goal attempts than Cleveland, which amounted to seven more opportunities per game. These factors affected the outcome prominently, especially in the game four and game six losses.

It should also be remembered that the O'Neal injury cost the team cohesiveness on the offensive side of the ball. Antawn Jamison arrived in a February trade just before Shaq injured his thumb. Mo Williams and Delonte West suffered injuries in January. On top of these factors, Mike Brown's coaching tactics during the Boston series were questioned not only by the media, but by his own players. A "ring for the king" turned into "gone for LeBron."

TREATMENT

The thumb has a strong, triangular-shaped ligament (ulnar collateral) near the base and it allows an athlete to grip objects (a baseball bat, basketball, ski pole, etc.). When the thumb is bent backward awkwardly, the ligament can stretch or tear (see medical illustration, page 306). In 1955, the term gamekeeper's thumb was used to describe this injury. As downhill skiing began to become more popular in the 1960s, injuries to the ulnar collateral ligament increased and were attributed to skiers breaking their falls with their poles, which stretched the thumb's ligaments. Medical professional began to call the injury skier's thumb.

In sports medicine, the thumb injury is seen frequently in ball-handling sports such as basketball. Severity of the injury is determined by a grading system.

- Grade 1 Sprain: a minor sprain with the ligament stretched but not torn. A grade 1 sprain can cause some range of motion (ROM) loss, swelling, and tenderness over the ligament.
- Grade 2 Sprain: a mild sprain with some ligament tearing. A grade 2 sprain can cause loss of ROM and grip strength.

- Grade 3 Sprain: A severe sprain with the ligament torn completely or a small piece of bone pulled off as the ligament separates from the bone. A grade 3 sprain can cause a total loss of function.

Treatment depends on several factors, including the extent of the injury and the physical demands of the patient. If the tear is partial, and the thumb is not too loose, the patient is usually placed in a cast or a modified wrist splint (spica splint) for up to six weeks. If the tear is complete, then surgery becomes more likely. Postoperatively, patients should wear a splint. In most cases, at three months after surgery, full activities can be resumed.

INCIDENTAL FINDINGS

Thumb injuries are not new. Materials for bandaging have been upgraded by technological advancements. However, techniques to immobilize a digit or limb were developed at the dawn of modern medicine.

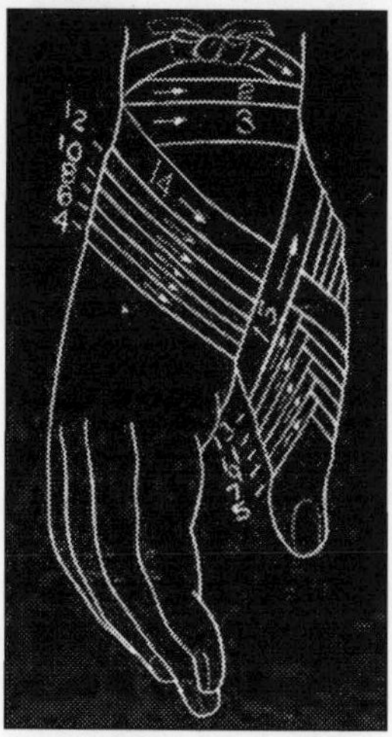
Spica of Thumb.

SPICA OF THE THUMB

Description—This bandage should be two yards in length by three-quarters of an inch in width.

Application—If it be the right you wish to bandage, place the hand midway between pronation and supination. Unroll four or five inches of the bandage, and thus place it, 1, upon the back of the wrist [see image], and confine by two circular turns, 2 and 3; continue in the same course till you come to the ulnar border of the hand, when you descend obliquely across the back of the hand to the radial side of the thumb, at the phalangeal articulation, thus finishing course 4. Pass under the thumb, and then up over it, and diagonally upwards to the radial side of the wrist, finishing course 5. Courses 6, 8, 10, 12 and 14, etc., respectively follow the course of turn 4; while those of 7, 9, 11, 13 and 15, those of course 5. At last exhaust the bandage by circular turns about the wrist, and confine by tying. (Henri Leonard, *Manual of Bandaging*, 6th ed., Detroit: Illustrated Medical Journal Co., 1884)

Appendix 1

Medical Illustrations

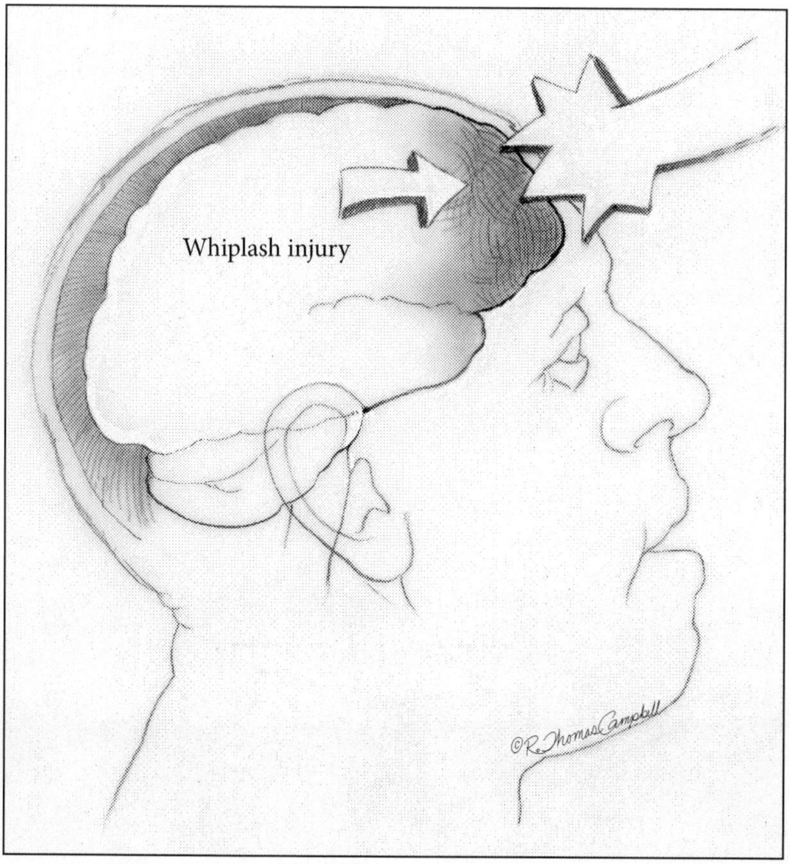

A blow to the head, leading to a rapid acceleration/deceleration of the brain in the cranial vault (skull), leading to brain injury (concussion). *Illustration by Thomas Campbell.*

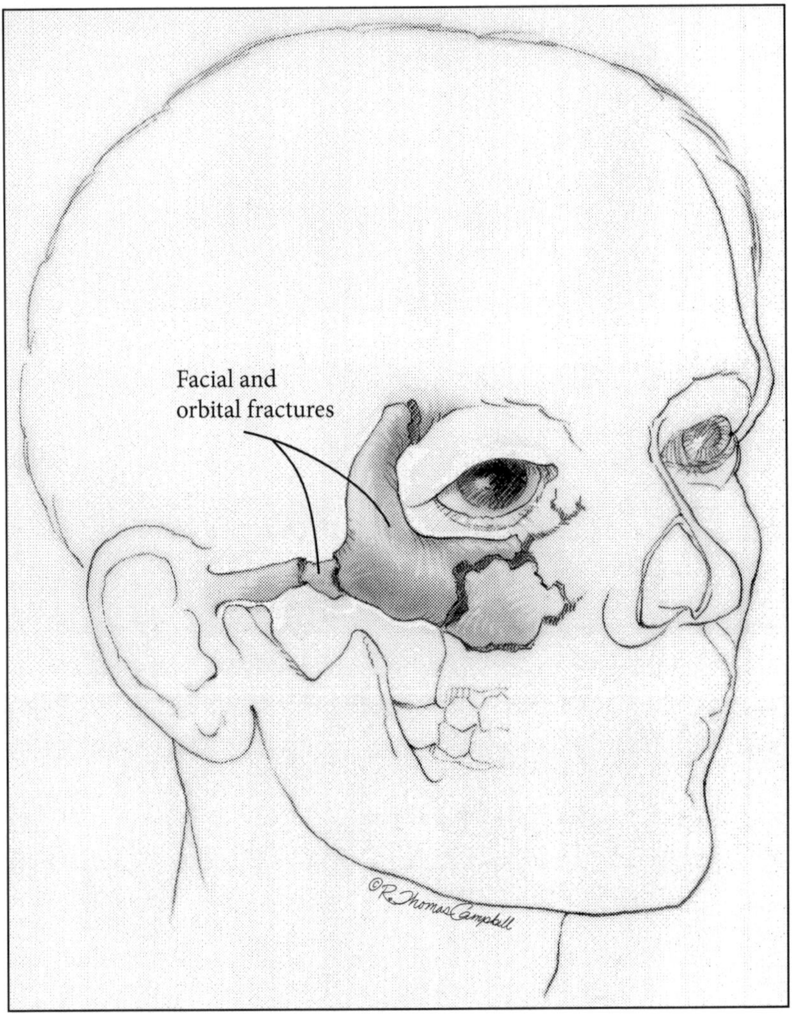

Facial and orbital fractures. *Illustration by Thomas Campbell.*

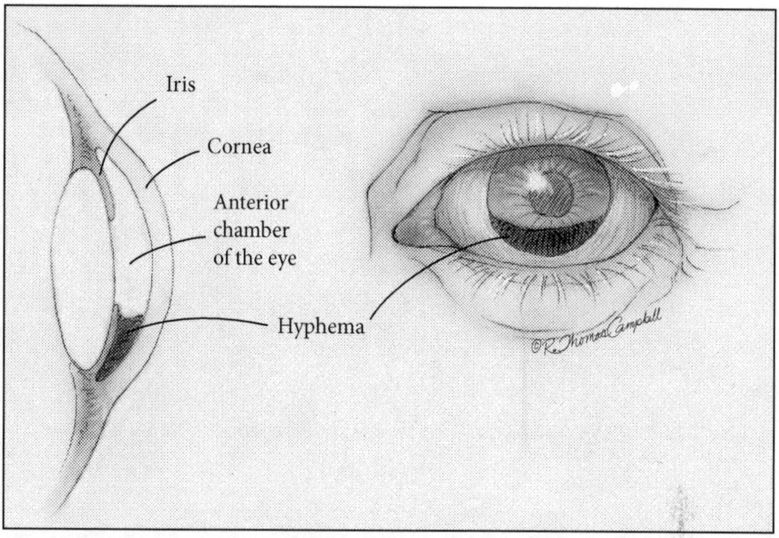

A hyphema, or blood, in the anterior chamber of the eye due to eye trauma.
Illustration by Thomas Campbell.

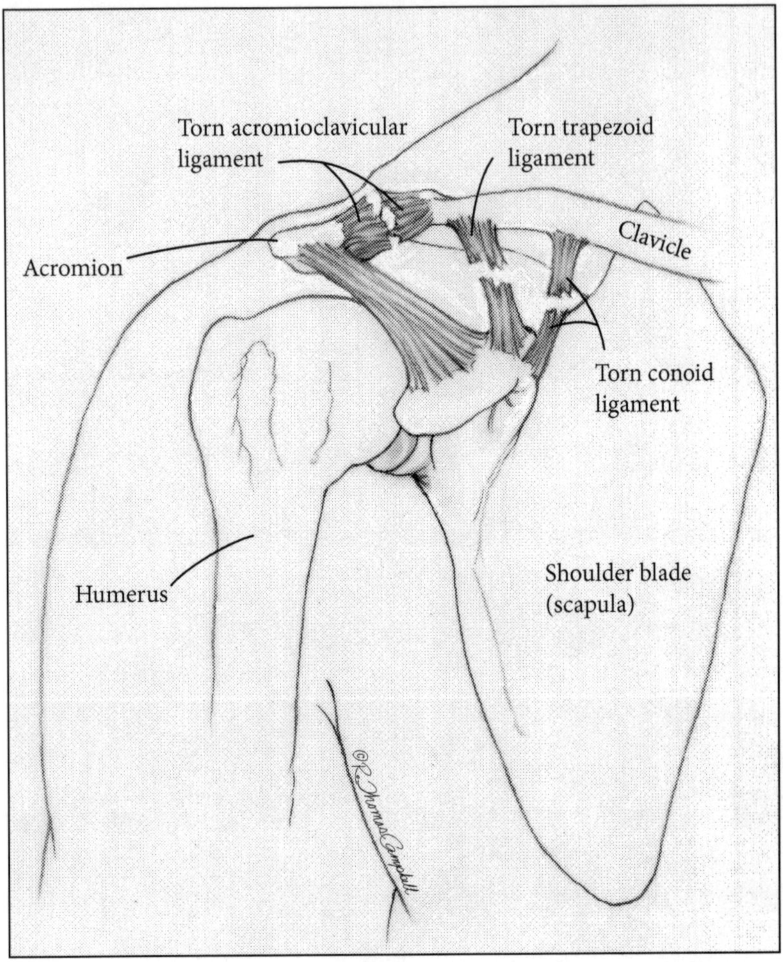

A tear to the ligaments supporting the acromioclavicular joint in the shoulder. This injury is known as a separated shoulder. *Illustration by Thomas Campbell.*

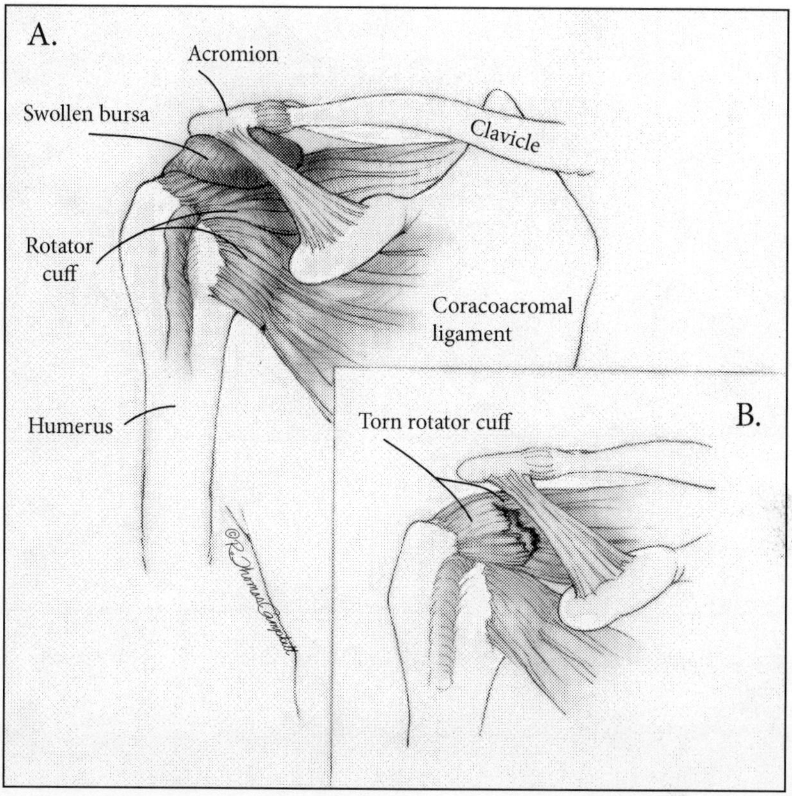

Swelling (inflammation) of the subacromial bursa, as seen in shoulder impingement (A). Advanced trauma to the subacromial space, resulting in a torn rotator cuff (B). *Illustration by Thomas Campbell.*

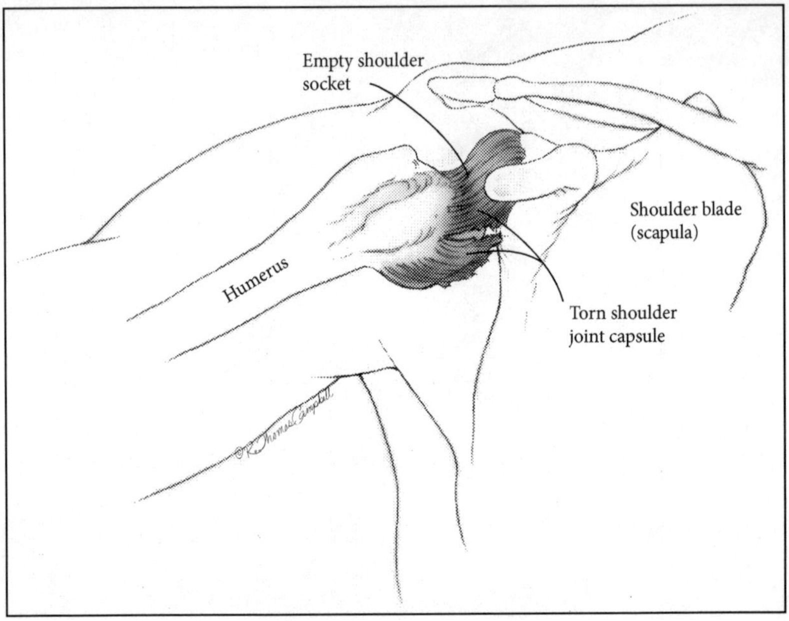

A torn shoulder capsule, resulting in a shoulder dislocation and empty socket. *Illustration by Thomas Campbell.*

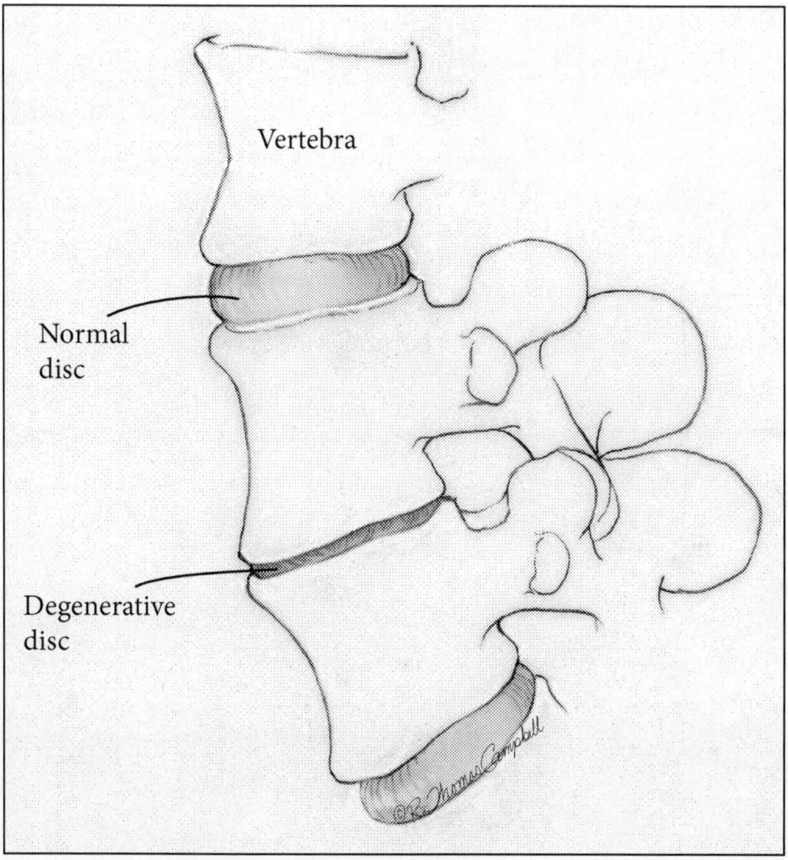

A narrowing of the disc space (degenerative disc) or worn-out shock absorber in the back. *Illustration by Thomas Campbell.*

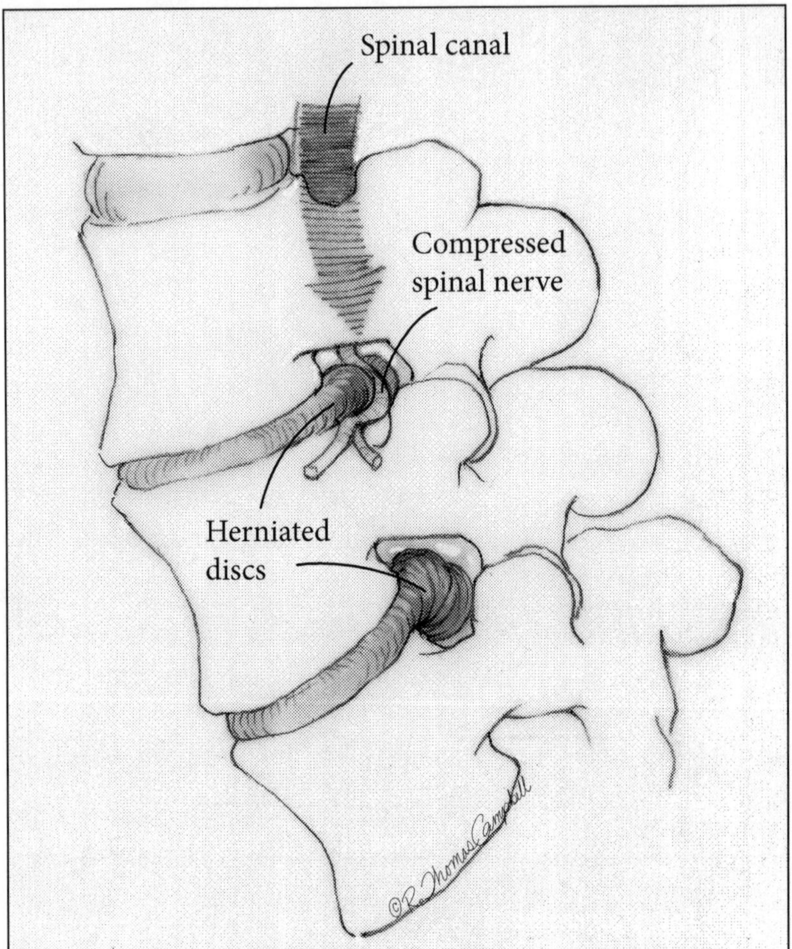

A slipped (herniated) disc, compressing the nerve route at two levels in the low back. *Illustration by Thomas Campbell.*

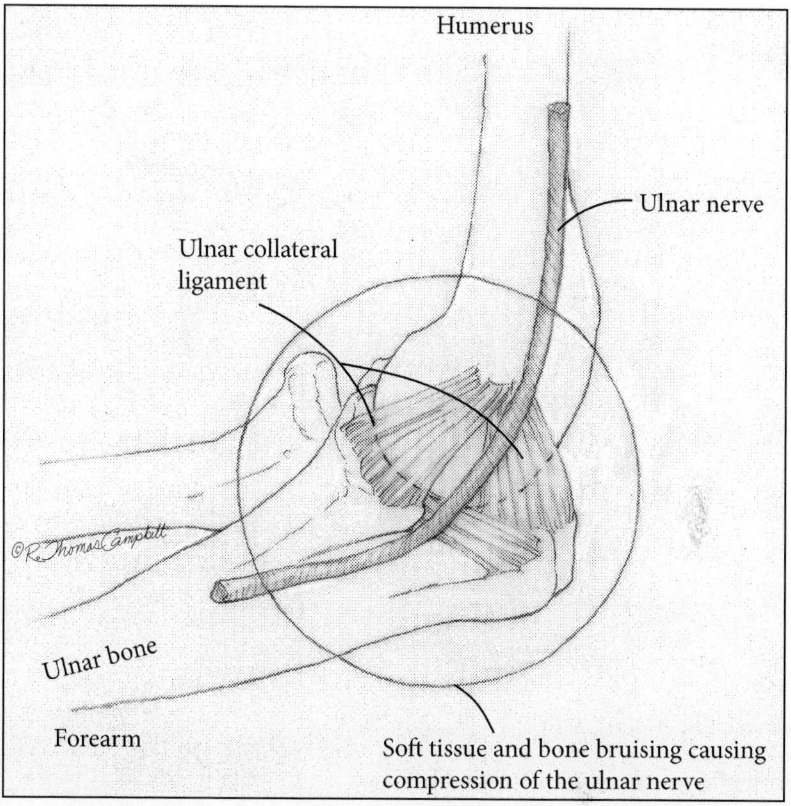

An entrapment (compression) of the ulnar nerve in the elbow. *Illustration by Thomas Campbell.*

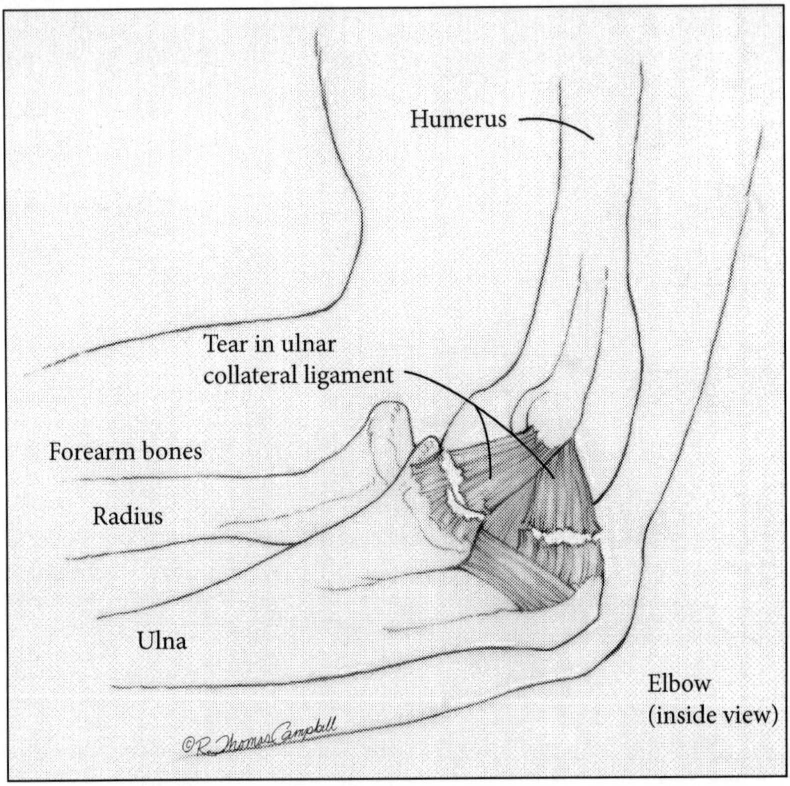

A tear in the triangular-shaped ulnar collateral ligament of the elbow. *Illustration by Thomas Campbell.*

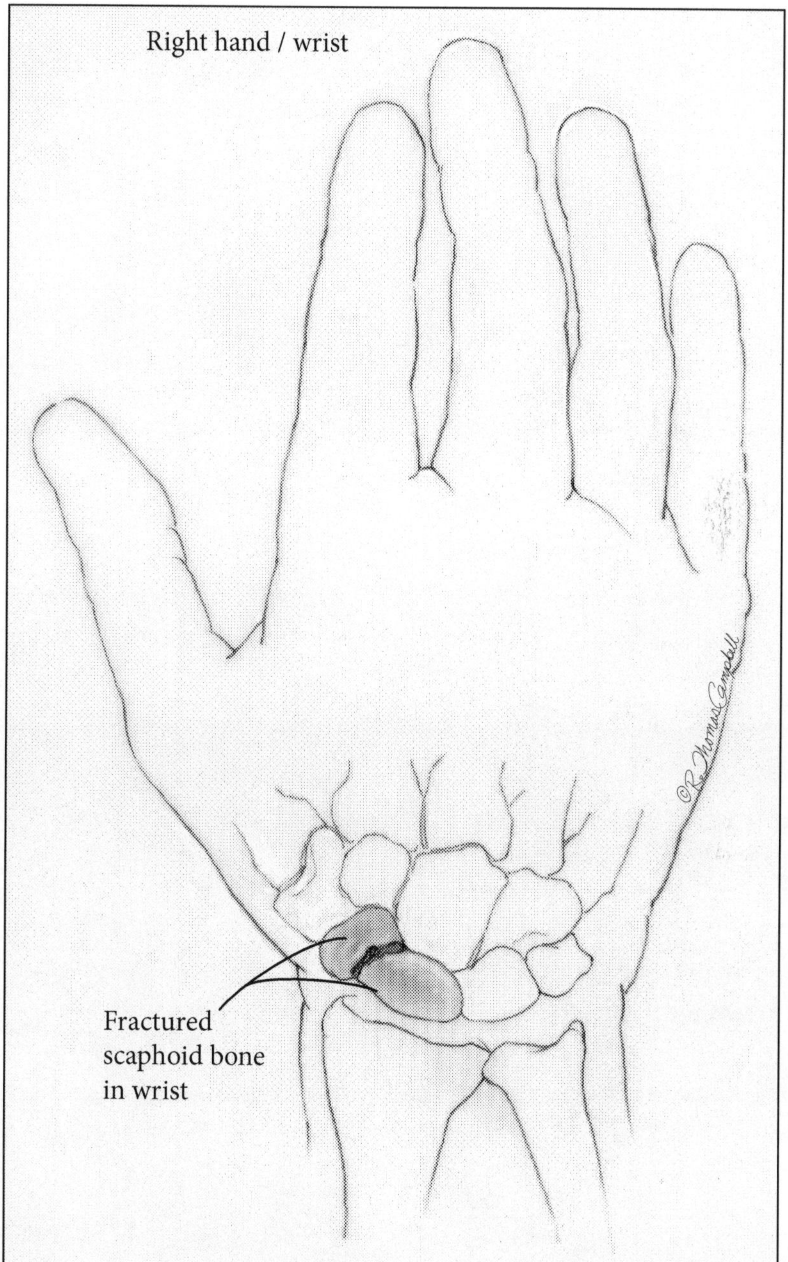

A fracture of the scaphoid (navicular) bone in the wrist. This injury occurs frequently from falls on an outstretched hand. *Illustration by Thomas Campbell.*

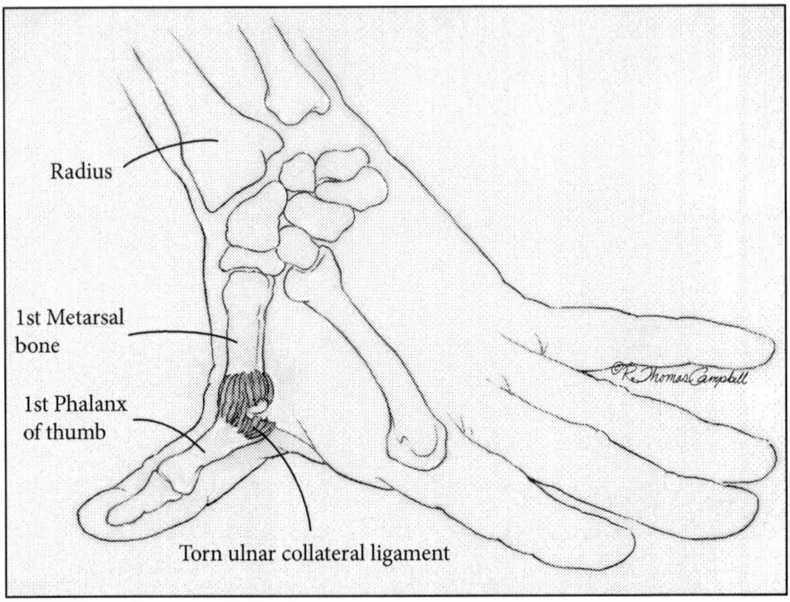

A partial tear of the ulnar collateral ligament in the thumb. *Illustration by Thomas Campbell.*

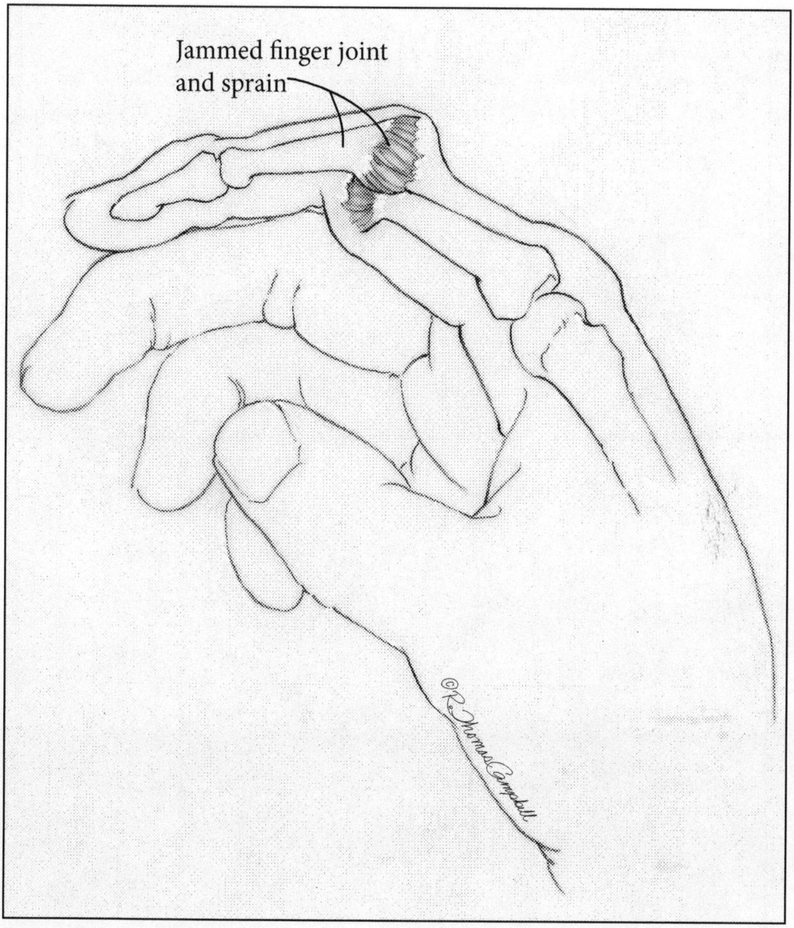

A torn ligament (sprain) of the middle joint (PIP) of the finger, resulting in a dislocation. This is the most common joint for a finger sprain and dislocation. *Illustration by Thomas Campbell.*

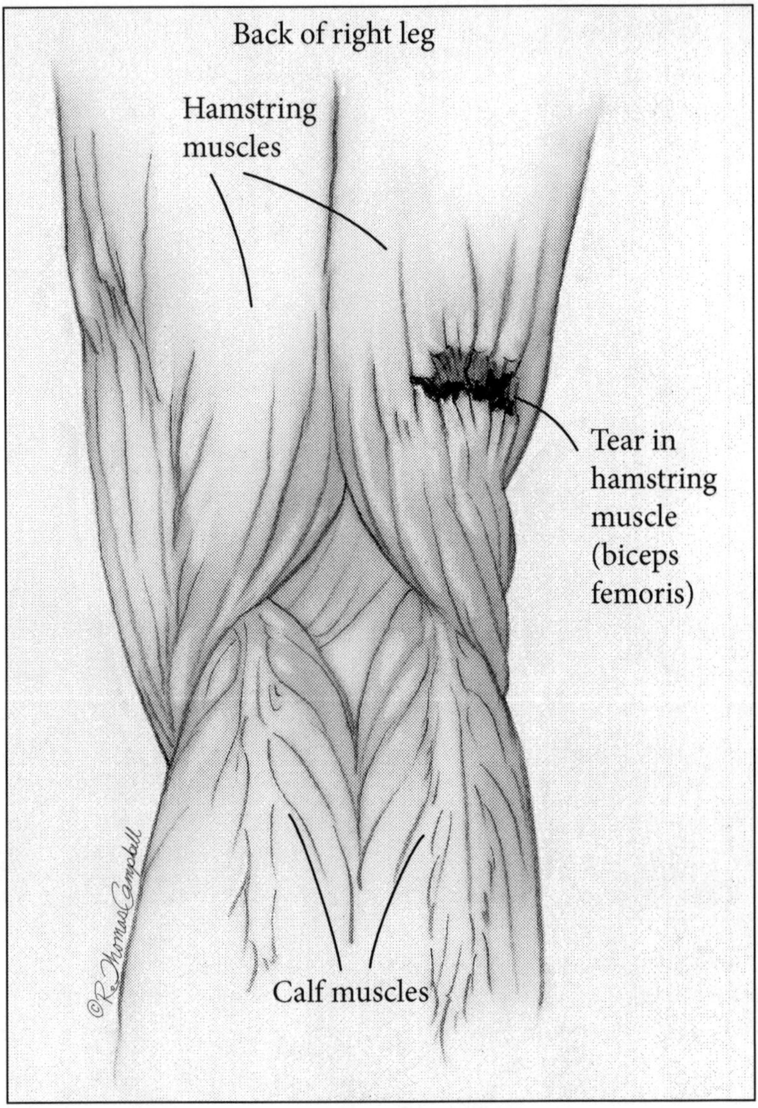

A hamstring tear, which occurs frequently in the lower hamstring where the muscle and tendon merge (muscle tendon junction). *Illustration by Thomas Campbell.*

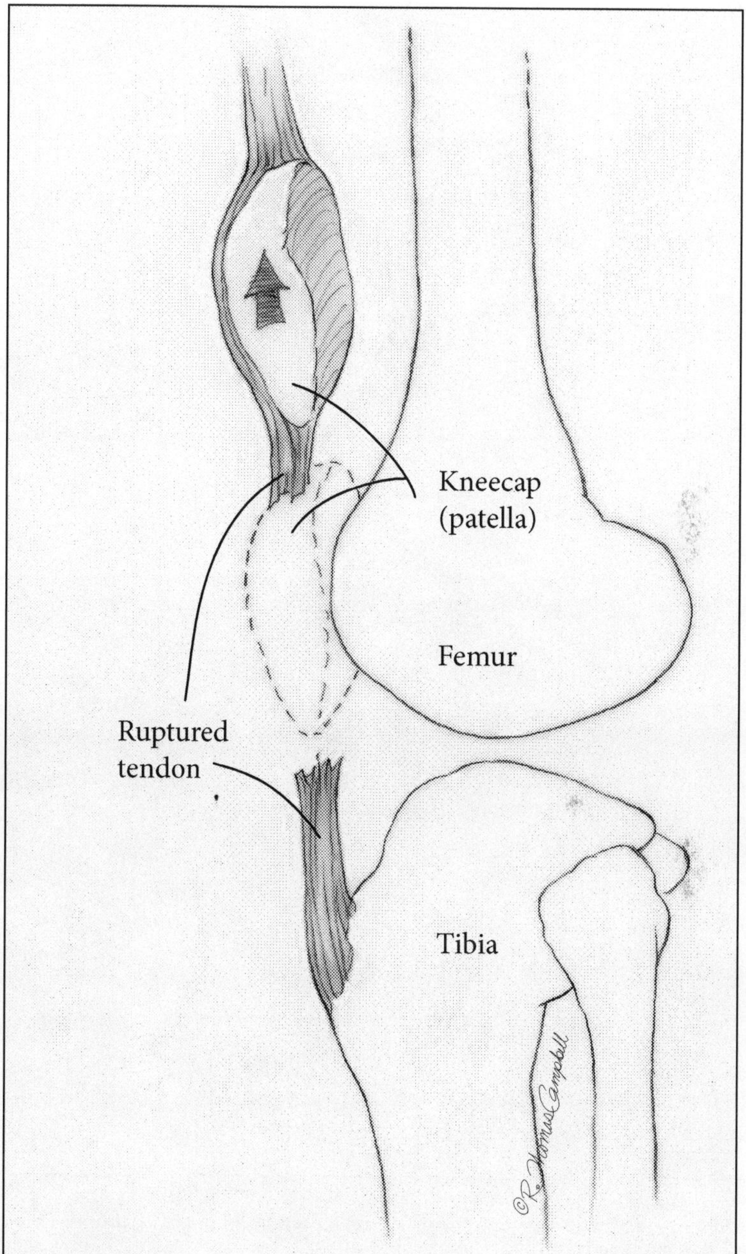

A tear or rupture in the infrapatellar tendon, leading to a retraction of the patella toward the hip. *Illustration by Thomas Campbell.*

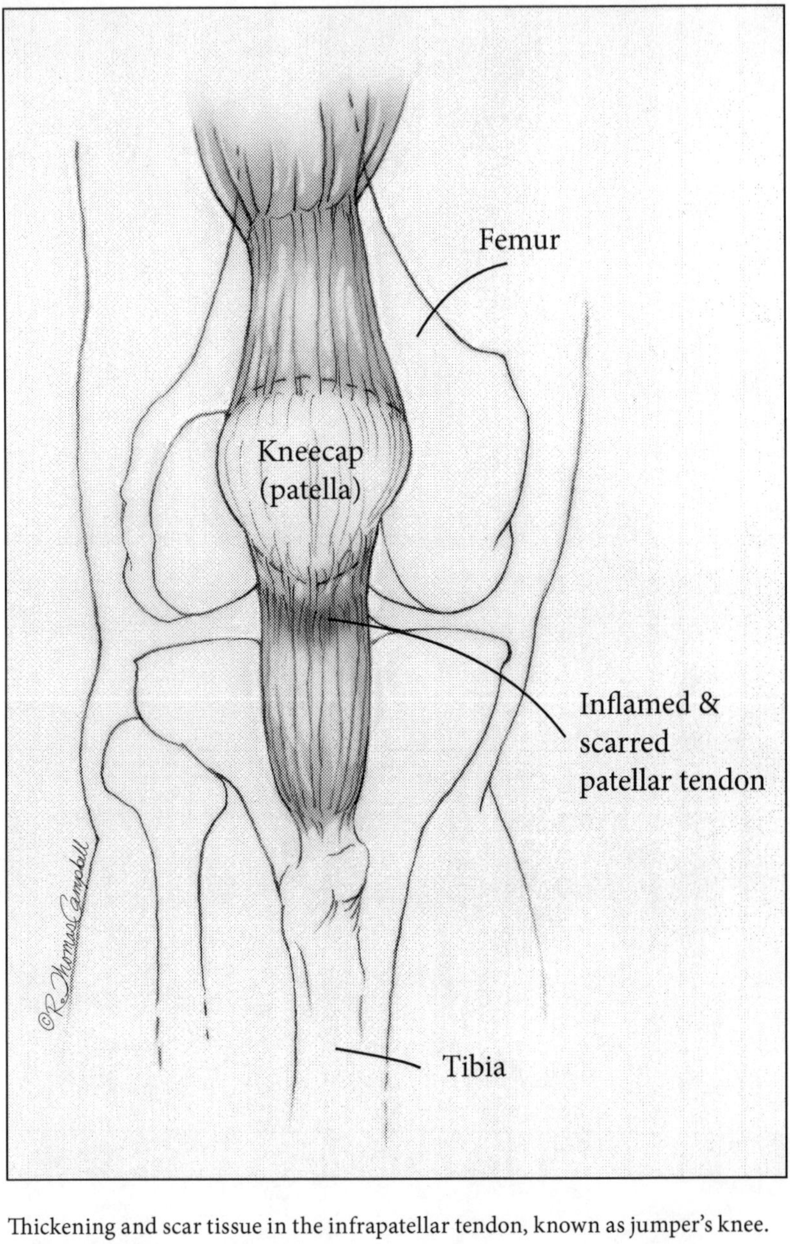

Thickening and scar tissue in the infrapatellar tendon, known as jumper's knee. *Illustration by Thomas Campbell.*

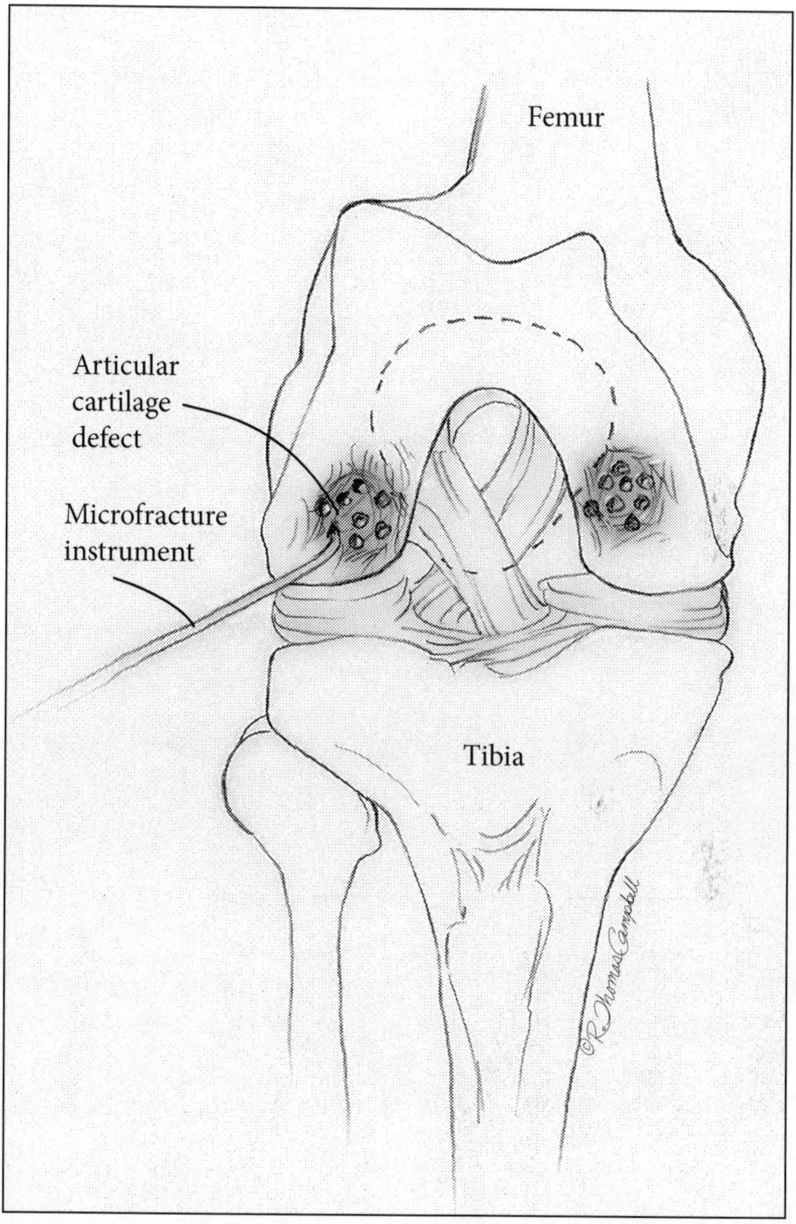

Microfracture surgery of the femur at the knee joint, which involves drilling a series of small holes into the articular cartilage to stimulate healing and new cartilage growth. *Illustration by Thomas Campbell.*

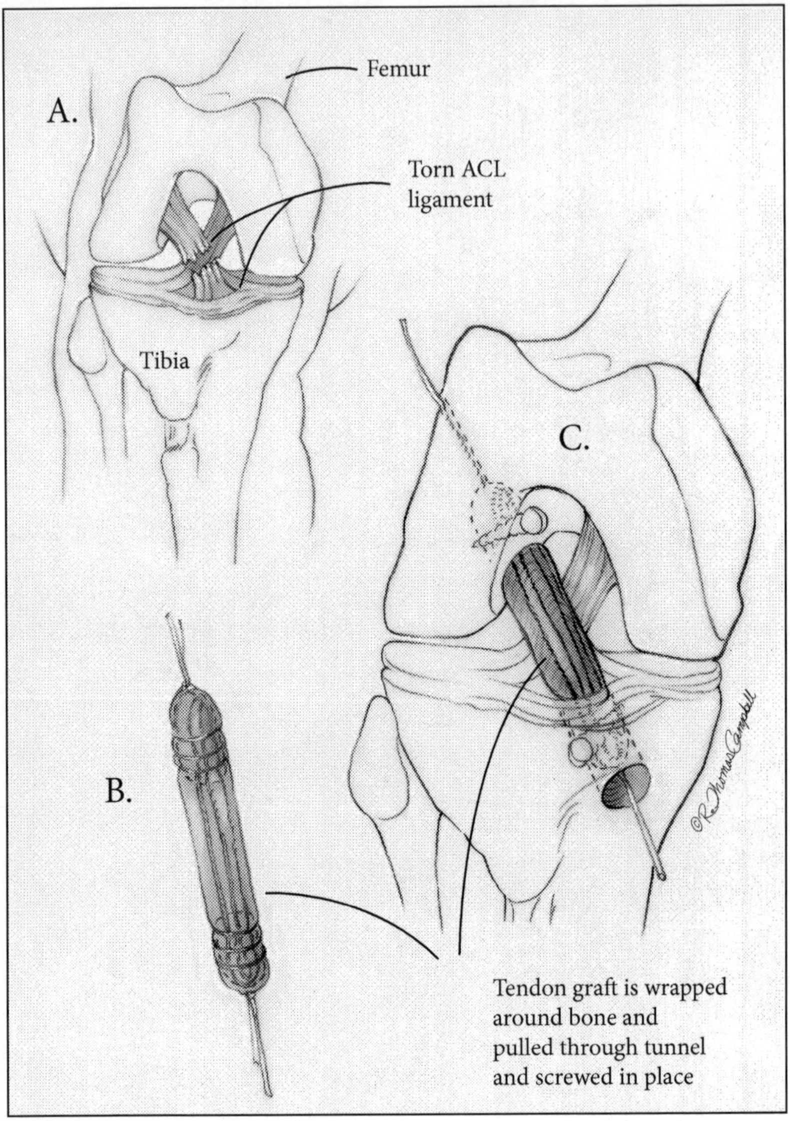

A rupture or tear (A) in the anterior cruciate ligament (ACL) and the use of a tendon graft to reconstruct a new ligament (B & C). *Illustration by Thomas Campbell.*

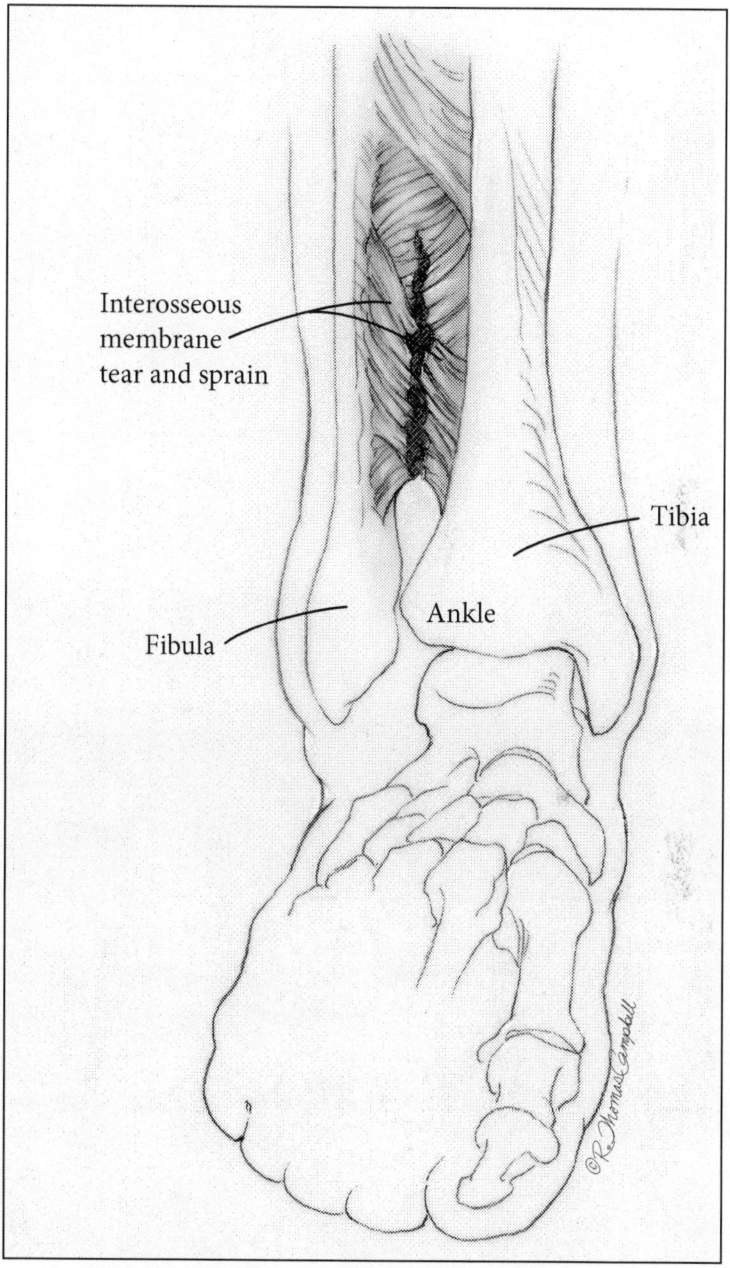

A torn tibiofibular ligament (syndesmosis and interosseous membrane) in the ankle, known as a high sprain. *Illustration by Thomas Campbell.*

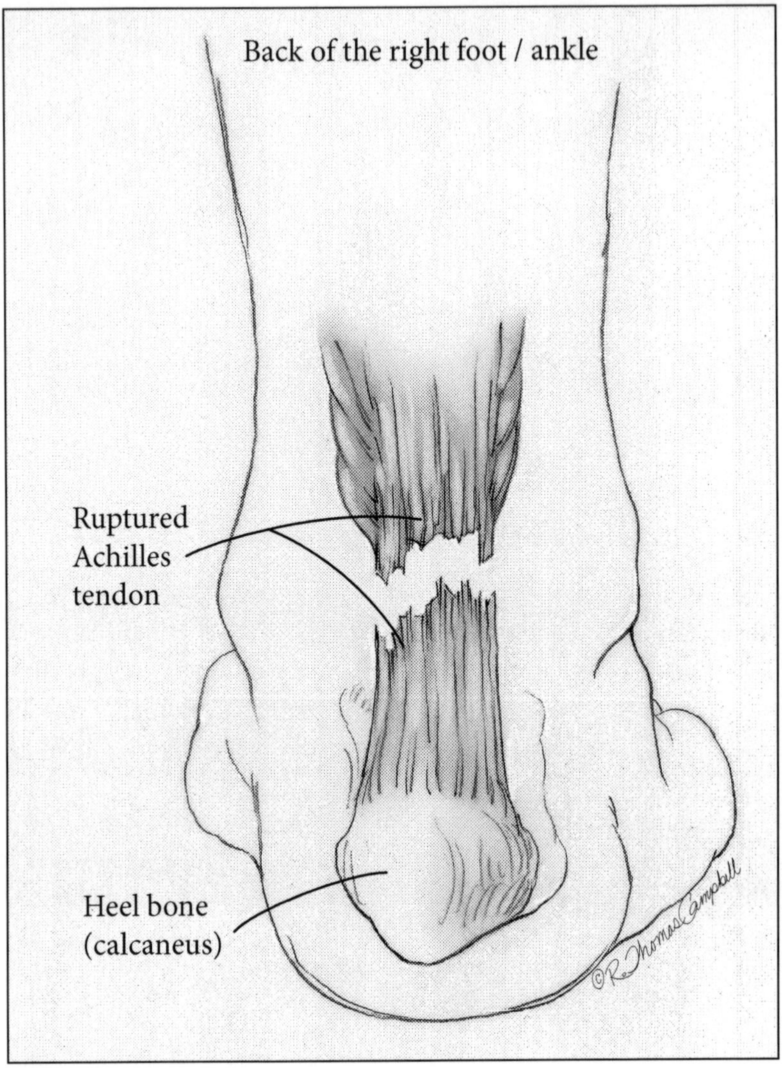

A rupture or tear of the Achilles' tendon. *Illustration by Thomas Campbell.*

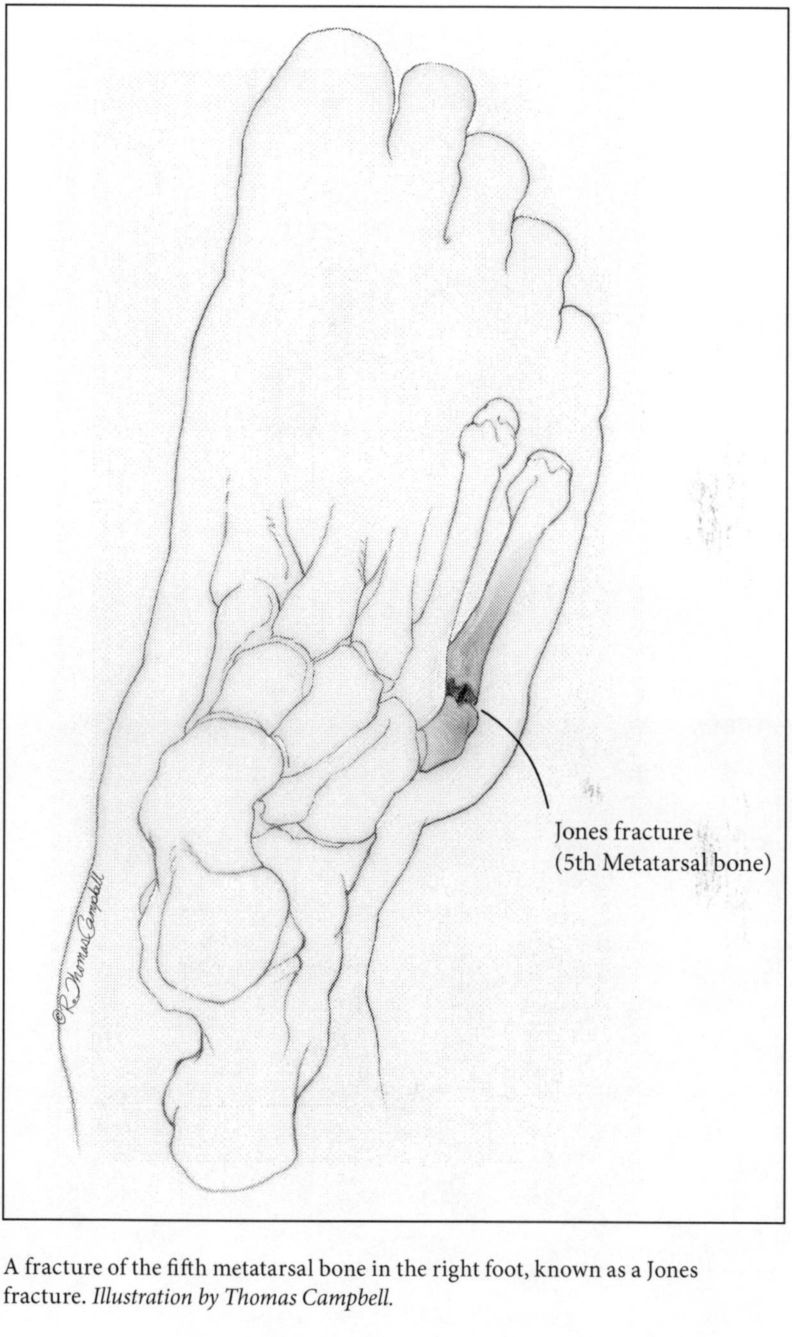

A fracture of the fifth metatarsal bone in the right foot, known as a Jones fracture. *Illustration by Thomas Campbell.*

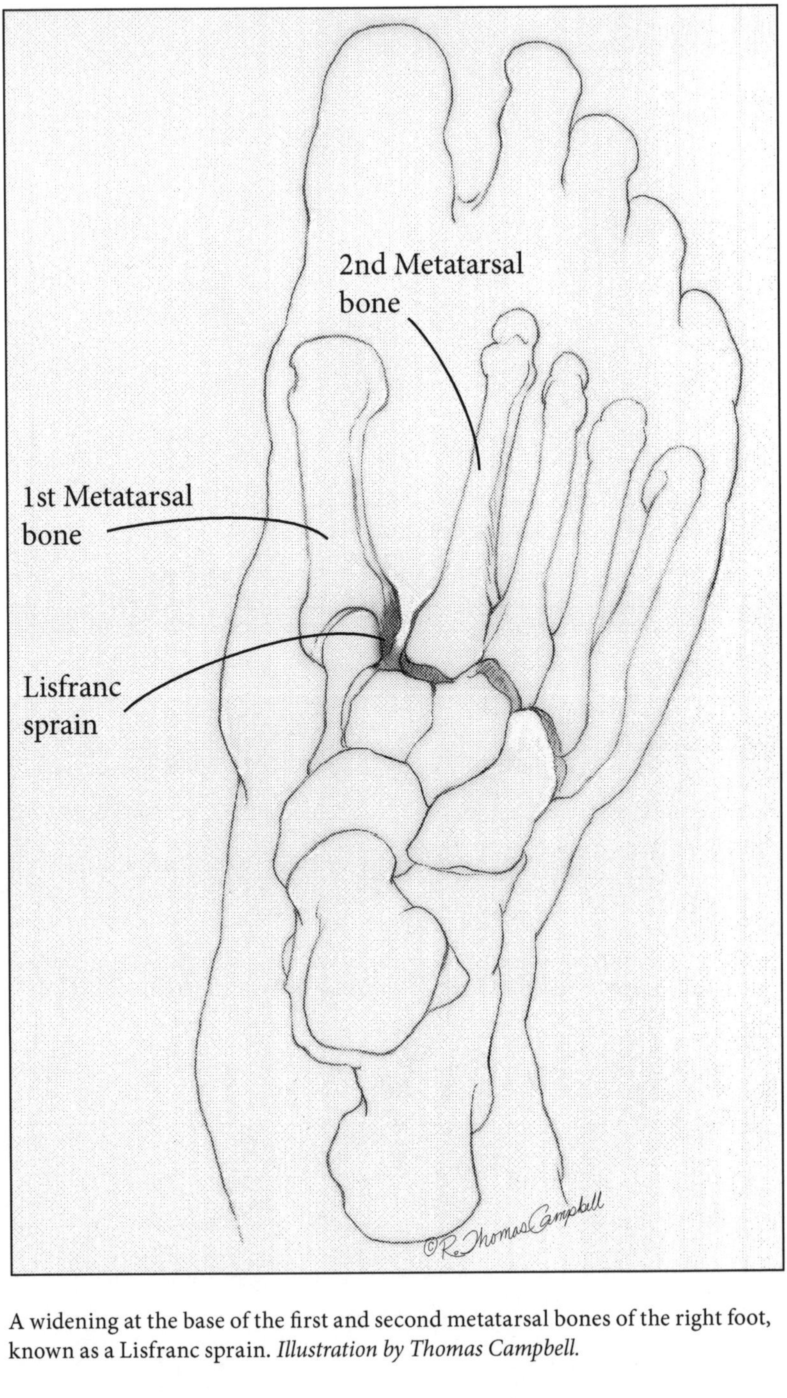

A widening at the base of the first and second metatarsal bones of the right foot, known as a Lisfranc sprain. *Illustration by Thomas Campbell.*

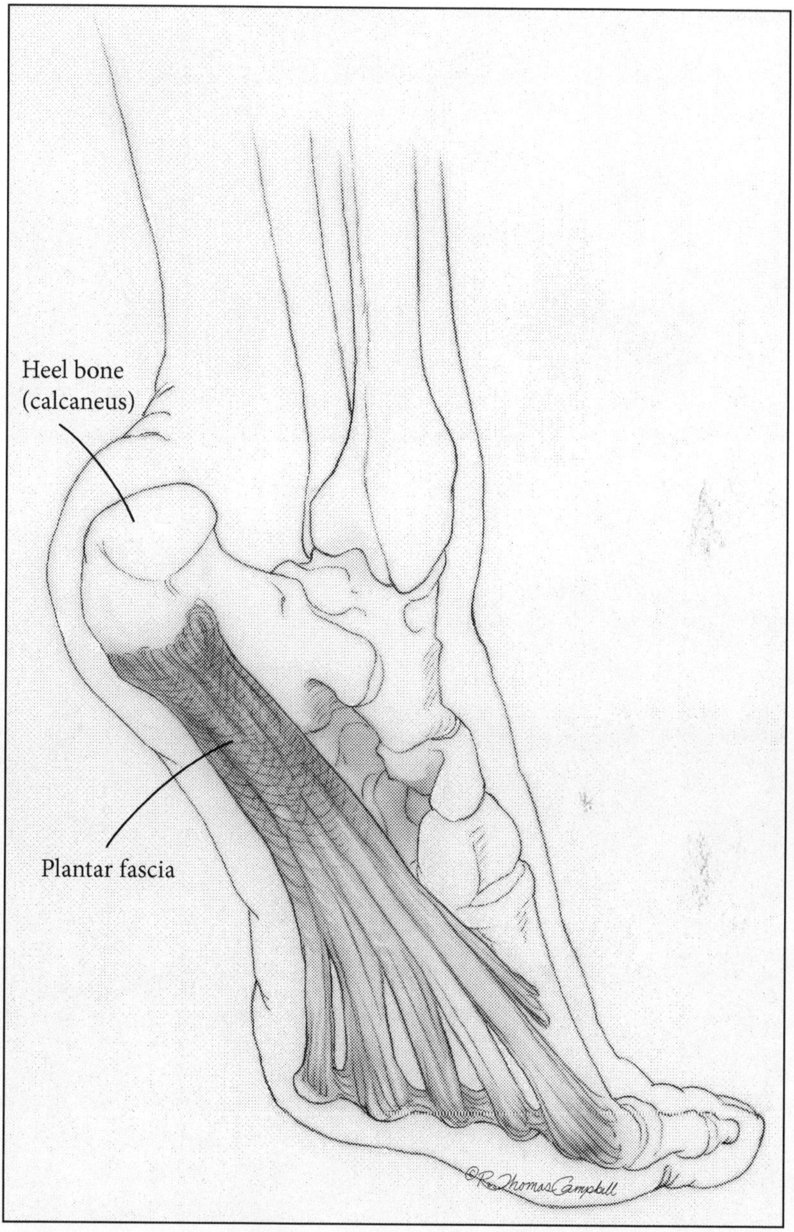

Thickening, scar tissue, and fibrosis, resulting in chronic plantar fasciitis.
Illustration by Thomas Campbell.

Appendix 2

Standardized Concussion Assessment Tool

Symptom Evaluation

How do you feel?

You should score yourself on the following symptoms, based on how you feel now.

	none	mild		moderate		severe	
Headache	0	1	2	3	4	5	6
"Pressure in head"	0	1	2	3	4	5	6
Neck Pain	0	1	2	3	4	5	6
Nausea or vomiting	0	1	2	3	4	5	6
Dizziness	0	1	2	3	4	5	6
Blurred vision	0	1	2	3	4	5	6
Balance problems	0	1	2	3	4	5	6
Sensitivity to light	0	1	2	3	4	5	6
Sensitivity to noise	0	1	2	3	4	5	6
Feeling slowed down	0	1	2	3	4	5	6
Feeling like "in a fog"	0	1	2	3	4	5	6
"Don't feel right"	0	1	2	3	4	5	6
Difficulty concentrating	0	1	2	3	4	5	6
Difficulty remembering	0	1	2	3	4	5	6
Fatigue or low energy	0	1	2	3	4	5	6
Confusion	0	1	2	3	4	5	6
Drowsiness	0	1	2	3	4	5	6
Trouble falling asleep (if applicable)	0	1	2	3	4	5	6
More emotional	0	1	2	3	4	5	6
Irritability	0	1	2	3	4	5	6
Sadness	0	1	2	3	4	5	6
Nervous or Anxious	0	1	2	3	4	5	6

Total number of symptoms (Maximum possible 22)

Symptom severity score

(Add all scores in table, maximum possible: 22 x 6 = 132)

Do the symptoms get worse with physical activity? Y N

Do the symptoms get worse with mental activity? Y N

Overall rating

If you know the athlete well prior to the injury, how different is the athlete acting compared to his / her usual self? Please circle one response.

no different	very different	unsure

Cognitive assessment

Standardized Assessment of Concussion (SAC)

Orientation (1 point for each correct answer)

What month is it?	0	1
What is the date today?	0	1
What is the day of the week?	0	1
What year is it?	0	1
What time is it right now? (within 1 hour)	0	1
Orientation score		of 5

Immediate memory

"I am going to test your memory. I will read you a list of words and when I am done, repeat back as many words as you can remember, in any order."

Trials 2 & 3:

"I am going to repeat the same list again. Repeat back as many words as you can remember in any order, even if you said the word before."

Complete all 3 trials regardless of score on trial 1 & 2. Read the words at a rate of one per second. Score 1 pt. for each correct response. Total score equals sum across all 3 trials. Do not inform the athlete that delayed recall will be tested.

List	Trial 1	Trial 2	Trial 3	Alternative word list		
elbow	0 1	0 1	0 1	candle	baby	finger
apple	0 1	0 1	0 1	paper	monkey	penny
carpet	0 1	0 1	0 1	sugar	perfume	blanket
saddle	0 1	0 1	0 1	sandwich	sunset	lemon
bubble	0 1	0 1	0 1	wagon	iron	insect
Total						

Immediate memory score of 15

Concentration

Digits Backward:

"I am going to read you a string of numbers and when I am done, you repeat them back to me backwards, in reverse order of how I read them to you. For example, if I say 7-1-9, you would say 9-1-7."

If correct, go to next string length. If incorrect, read trial 2. One point possible for each string length. Stop after incorrect on both trials. The digits should be read at the rate of one per second.

			Alternative digit lists		
4-9-3	0	1	6-2-9	5-2-6	4-1-5
3-8-1-4	0	1	3-2-7-9	1-7-9-5	4-9-6-8
6-2-9-7-1	0	1	1-5-2-8-6	3-8-5-2-7	6-1-8-4-3
7-1-8-4-6-2	0	1	5-3-9-1-4-8	8-3-1-9-6-4	7-2-4-8-5-6

Months in Reverse Order:

"Now tell me the months of the year in reverse order. Start with the last month and go backward. So you'll say December, November ... Go ahead"

1 pt. for entire sequence correct

Dec-Nov-Oct-Sept-Aug-Jul-Jun-May-Apr-Mar-Feb-Jan	0	1
Concentration score		

Sideline Assessment – Maddocks Score

"I am going to ask you a few questions, please listen carefully and give your best effort."

Modified Maddocks questions (1 point for each correct answer)

At what venue are we at today?	0	1
Which half is it now?	0	1
Who scored last in this match?	0	1
What team did you play last week/game?	0	1
Did your team win the last game?	0	1

Maddocks score of 5

Maddocks score is validated for sideline diagnosis of concussion only and is not included in SCAT 2 summary score for serial testing.

Cognitive assessment

Standardized Assessment of Concussion (SAC)

Delayed recall

"Do you remember that list of words I read a few times earlier? Tell me as many words from the list as you can remember in any order."

Circle each word correctly recalled. Total score equals number of words recalled.

List	Alternative word list		
elbow	candle	baby	finger
apple	paper	monkey	penny
carpet	sugar	perfume	blanket
saddle	sandwich	sunset	lemon
bubble	wagon	iron	insect

Delayed recall score of 5